Praise for
All Together Healthy
A Canadian Wellness Revolution

"Well researched, clear and convincing. *All Together Healthy* makes a strong case for improving our healthcare system by outlining the social factors that comprise wellbeing. The more we think 'together' the healthier we'll be—sings the wellness revolution."

— Raffi Cavoukian, singer, author, founder of Child Honouring

"*All Together Healthy* makes the compelling case that poor health is caused by societal factors such as income inequality and lack of investment in early childhood. MacLeod combines story-telling and evidence in a passionate and timely call for all of us to rethink our conception of and approach to health and to participate in building the much healthier society we could be."

— Monika Dutt, M.D., Executive Director of Upstream
and past chair of Canadian Doctors for Medicare

"Andrew MacLeod has created a masterpiece that reflects universal influences on human health, illustrating how our health is impacted by broad social patterns, especially social marginalization. This inspiring book is a compelling argument against empty, self-interested rhetoric, and for enacting real, comprehensive and intelligently informed kindness towards all citizens, in order to lift up society as a whole."

— Warren Bell, family physician and past founding president of
the Canadian Association of Physicians for the Environment

ALL TOGETHER HEALTHY

A Canadian Wellness Revolution

ANDREW MACLEOD

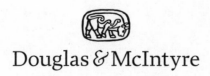

Douglas & McIntyre

Douglas and McIntyre (2013) Ltd.
P.O. Box 219, Madeira Park, BC, VON 2H0
www.douglas-mcintyre.com

Edited by Pam Robertson
Indexed by Nicola Goshulak
Cover design by Setareh Ashrafologhalai
Text design by Shed Simas / Onça Design
Printed and bound in Canada

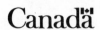 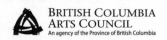 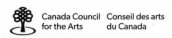

Douglas and McIntyre (2013) Ltd. acknowledges the support of the Canada Council
for the Arts, which last year invested $153 million to bring the arts to Canadians
throughout the country. We also gratefully acknowledge financial support from the
Government of Canada and from the Province of British Columbia through the BC
Arts Council and the Book Publishing Tax Credit.

Library and Archives Canada Cataloguing in Publication

MacLeod, Andrew, 1972-, author
    All together healthy : a Canadian wellness revolution / Andrew MacLeod.

Includes bibliographical references and index.
Issued in print and electronic formats.
ISBN 978-1-77162-188-5 (softcover).--ISBN 978-1-77162-189-2 (HTML)

    1. Health--Social aspects--Canada. 2. Medical policy--Canada.
I. Title.

RA395.C3M29 2018   306.4'610971   C2018-900875-X
                                                 C2018-900876-8

To my parents

"Historians tell us that we have had two great revolutions in the course of public health ... The third revolution, in which governments and citizens work together to address the determinants of health, will ensure that Candians are the healthiest we can be."

— Roy Romanow, foreword to *A Healthy Society*[1]

"It seemed to me then—it sometimes seems to me now, for that matter—that economic injustice will stop the moment we want it to stop, and no sooner, and if we genuinely want it to stop the method adopted hardly matters."

— George Orwell, *The Road to Wigan Pier*

Contents

Introduction   9

1 **Chronic Illness**   13
Little Care for a Known
Problem

2 **Diagnosis**   33
Health Care and Canadian
Pride

3 **Bad Habits**   45
Wasteful Spending and
Ignored Needs

4 **Causes of the Causes**   63
Living Conditions, Wealth
and Status

5 **Worrying Symptoms**   79
Mental Health Care and
Tent Cities

6 **Self-Medicating**   95
The Overdose Crisis and
Untreated Trauma

7 **Healing Traditions**   112
Trauma, Land and
Indigenous Health

8 **Environmental Risk**   134
Climate Change, Pollution
and Togetherness

9 **Healthy Beginnings**   145
Childhood and Future
Hopes

10 **Treatment**   164
Supporting Incomes and
Broad Approaches

11 **Prevention**   176
Persistent Blockages and
Sunny Ways

12 **Better**   188
Acting Together for
Healthy Generations

Endnotes   195
Acknowledgments   219
Select Bibliography   221
Index   231
About the Author   240

Introduction

When I was a child, my father ran a laboratory at the Hospital for Sick Children in downtown Toronto. One day when I was about twelve, a friend and I were left to explore the lab while we waited for my dad to finish some work. With a piece of rubber tube, we hooked a glass filtering flask up to the lab's vacuum system. I put the wide, open mouth of the bottle against my cheek. It formed a tight seal, pulling a circle of flesh into the bottle as the vacuum intensified. It began to hurt. A lot. There was some fumbling with the lever that controlled the vacuum, and we may have turned the pressure up instead of off. I tugged hard on the flask and it came off my cheek with a loud pop. Soon a dark, perfectly circular bruise rose on my face. "What I demonstrated," I joked at my dad's retirement dinner many years later, "is that while curiosity may be genetic, clearly intelligence is not."

My mother also worked in health care. A physiotherapist, for many years she worked on a palliative care unit helping as people approached death. At her own retirement party, she advocated that it was time to "blow up the system and let the healers emerge." The remark was met with uncomfortable titters from some of the colleagues she was leaving, but what she was getting at is that in health care there are many services that are provided because they always have been. People with entrenched interests were at times more interested in protecting their turf than they were in allowing innovation. While people would always need care, there are many ways to provide it.

My dad was remarried many years ago to a woman who has a PhD in pharmacology and who organized clinical trials for a drug company. In both homes, medical topics predominated and for a while I thought I might follow into the field. From when I was little, working in medicine had seemed a good idea. The family car had a licence plate that started

MDD, which my dad said would be a signal to police if there'd been an accident that he could help. Before reaching school age I often dug into my father's black medical bag and played with the otoscope for looking in ears, his stethoscope and the reflex hammer. With the tools spread out on the carpet before me, there seemed no better calling than to have the skills to help when people are sick or injured.

Somewhere along the way my plans shifted. I entered university describing myself as a pre-med student, took science courses, but found the memorization in chemistry and biology classes a chore. I was more interested in participating on the school newspaper, where the stated and overly self-serious ambition to be "agents of social change" appealed. I took a year out of studying to co-edit the paper and when I went back to the classroom it was to take courses in English, history, philosophy and other arts. After graduating I found work as a reporter and over two decades I've written frequently about health, poverty, social issues and the environment. While writing thousands of stories I've had a chance to see up close the role public policy could play in improving the health of many people. Journalism has turned out to be a way to stay near the family business without having to mind the shop, as the saying goes.

This book, and the idiosyncratic path it takes, is the result of that interest. It is about how to maximize the health of the maximum number of people. As the World Health Organization's constitution defines it, "Health is a state of complete physical, mental and social well-being and not merely the absence of disease or infirmity."[1] Is encouraging good health then a matter of paying for the newest drugs and latest hospital technology, or are there better options? Are there more gains to be had through stem cell research and gene therapy, or by addressing the conditions in which families raise children, which are linked to the risk of depression, diabetes, heart disease and a host of conditions? While poverty and its effects are part of the story, they are not the full story. If everyone were as healthy as the country's top income earners, there would be significantly fewer deaths each year. About half of the avoidable deaths come from the poorest group, but the other half come from the middle groups, making the damaging effects of inequity something that should be of concern to people all the way up the income ladder.

Rooted on Canada's west coast, this book considers policy choices that are made at the national and provincial levels. In Canada, it's provinces and territories that manage not only the health care systems, but also education, welfare and other relevant programs. And the effects are seen locally. There may be an international trend towards smaller governments and weaker social supports, but that shift is most visible when a line-up gathers at the local food bank or a tent city sprouts in a downtown park. Still, this book draws on research from other countries and looks outward so that it's clear how the observations apply more broadly. It is about health, public policy and steps we can take together.

As the politicians like to say, we are at a critical juncture that will determine our future. In Canada, as in many other countries, we have had three decades largely characterized by government austerity and growing inequality. That social inequity manifests in health inequities. But the public discussion tends to ignore that many of the prime determinants of a person's health lie outside the individual's immediate control. We're told to eat our vegetables, get a good sleep and avoid smoking. When something goes wrong, thankfully, there's the health care system.

The health care system has a role, and it's worth examining what it does well and where it falls short. It should not, however, be allowed to dominate the debate and demands for funding the way it does in Canada and the United States. More attention needs to be given to other factors. Education, employment, housing, the natural environment and social supports—particularly for families with children—also have great impacts on the health of individuals and our communities. So do social status and income, which is in fact the top indicator of how healthy an individual is likely to be.

For Canada and several provinces, we are in a moment of political optimism where other paths seem possible, but it is uncertain what path will be chosen and whether promised changes will happen. My hope is to define what's at stake and articulate a goal that gives priority to supporting our general well-being and good health. To create the world we want, first we must imagine it.

CHAPTER 1

Chronic Illness

Little Care for a
Known Problem

Good health would seem to be a widely shared obsession. Magazine racks and newspapers overflow with advice on how to boost your energy, shrink your belly, renew your body and look great naked. You should walk more, practise safer sex and avoid smoking, the articles tell us. Get out of your chair, build a standing desk and walk on a treadmill while working. Eat a rainbow of vegetables. Get enough sleep. If you fail to follow the advice, well, you've made your choice. Though prevalent, it's a perspective that ignores decades of evidence that most of what determines a person's health is beyond the individual's control. It individualizes the problem, implying that if you are fat, diabetic or sick, it's your own fault.

The message that health is solely an individual responsibility is reinforced by the disease advocacy groups. The Heart and Stroke Foundation of Canada counsels that "Up to 80% of premature heart disease and stroke can be prevented" and offers tips on diet, exercise and stress on its website. "In the mistaken idea that it will make them feel better, some people react to stress by turning to unhealthy habits, such as eating high-fat comfort foods, smoking, excessive alcohol consumption or overeating." Best to avoid stress in the first place, it says, advising you to know what stresses you out, find ways to cope and "get rid of stress daily." Its suggestions for eating out are particularly detailed:

At the restaurant, opt for a whole-grain offering from the bread-basket as opposed to higher-fat, buttery garlic bread. Many appetizers are deep-fried or high in fat and calories, so choose a vegetable-based soup or a dark, leafy green salad with dressing on the side. Order an entrée that is described as baked, barbe-cued, broiled, charbroiled, grilled, poached, roasted, steamed or stir-fried. Avoid dishes with the words Alfredo sauce, au gra-tin, cheese sauce, battered, breaded, buttered, creamed, crispy, deep-fried, en croute, fried, hollandaise, pan-fried, pastry, prime, rich, sautéed, scalloped, gravy, mayonnaise or thick sauce, as it usually means the dish is higher in fat and calories. If going to a fast food restaurant, look online or at the restaurant for nutritional information. Comparing the calories, fat and sodium content can help you make the best choice possible.[1]

Reading the advice, even though following it would no doubt be wise, I'm reminded of an old joke: by cutting out rich food, cigarettes and alcohol you may not live longer, but at least your life will *feel* longer.

The website for another group, Diabetes Canada, promotes diet, nutrition, exercise and managing your weight. It includes lifestyle tips and makes clear who it sees as responsible: "Taking care of your health should be your top priority."

There is, however, abundant evidence that type two diabetes, which accounts for 90 percent of cases, is closely tied to income. As Dennis Raphael, who is a health policy and management professor at York University in Toronto, put it in a phone interview, "Even if poor people exercised and their weight was in the so-called 'normal' range, they'd still be two to three times more likely to get diabetes." And yet a search of the Diabetes Canada website for the word "poverty" returns just one docu-ment, a press release noting that Nova Scotia's 2017 budget included $2 million to begin addressing poverty.[2] There's little acknowledgment that at each step down the income ladder the chances a person will become diabetic increase (see Figure 1.1).

Pronouncements about choice and lifestyle are standard fare for governments as well. British Columbia's 2005 throne speech had "five goals for a golden decade" that included "Make B.C. a model for healthy

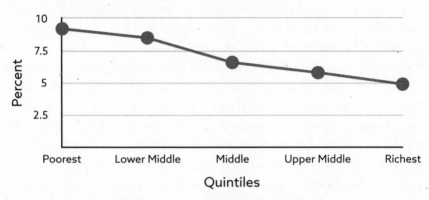

Fig 1.1   Diabetes Prevalence by Income Quintile

Source   Statistics Canada, Canadian Community Health Survey

living and physical fitness." Ontario maintains a "healthy choices" website that instructs citizens on "how to make choices for a healthy life" and includes tips on healthy eating, food safety, hand washing and active living.[3] Making healthier choices will make you feel better, reduce stress and prevent diseases, it promises. The Québec en Forme program is a partnership between the provincial government and the Lucie and André Chagnon Foundation to promote healthy eating and active living for families.[4]

Federally, the Canadian government has for generations provided a food guide promoting healthy eating and funded campaigns to encourage physical fitness.[5] Health Canada's website acknowledges that some choices may be restricted by an individual's circumstances, but ultimately suggests those too are a matter of choice themselves. "Healthy living choices are affected by where you live, work, learn and play. Keeping yourself informed about positive health practices within your environment is an important way to improve your overall health and sense of well-being." The underlying premise is that knowing more about what contributes to good health is the first step towards achieving it.

The problem is that for most people, for most diseases, knowledge isn't enough. Staying up to the minute on all the latest health information is daunting and may not provide the hoped-for benefits. A professor of law and public health in Edmonton, Timothy Caulfield wrote about his experience trying to put all the latest research into practice in his 2012 book *The Cure for Everything.* "For the year that I worked on this book I completely submerged myself in the world of health science," he wrote. "I exercised like a maniac, went on an ultra-healthy diet, got my genes tested, and tried a variety of remedies. It was a fascinating journey that led to some surprising conclusions about what the science actually says and the degree to which this message gets twisted." Despite that diligent effort, which was far more than most people would be willing or able to make, Caulfield found it failed to make a noticeable difference to his health. "The results of my research point to a disheartening conclusion, which is, basically, that nothing works. Despite the immense diet, fitness, and remedy industries, very little actually does what it promises to do."[6]

Being nagged by the prime minister or anyone else won't help either. Nor will a smartphone in every pocket, a Fitbit on every wrist or a pedometer on every belt make a large-scale difference. It might help a few committed individuals become healthier, but there are better, more likely, ways to improve the health of the population as a whole. In some cases, as we'll see, the nagging has actually made health inequities wider. Everyone knows, for example, that smoking is bad for them, but some people are significantly more able than others to avoid or break the habit.

There are much larger forces underlying the choices individuals make that have a much stronger effect on how healthy we are as a people. Often described as the "social determinants of health," these forces play out across populations, providing an answer to the question of why some people appear to make worse choices than others, and pointing towards why some people are healthier than others.

Take the example of J. Gary Pelerine, who at fifty-eight years old had for a year been fighting cancer that had first appeared on his tongue. It was only his latest setback. "You got no idea what my luck's been like in my life. Of course I've got cancer," he said. He'd recently dropped thirty-five pounds due to the illness and was fighting to get the government to add a nutritional supplement to the disability assistance money he received. Over the course of an hour he smoked several cigarettes. None of the medical people had linked the cancer to smoking, a pleasure he'd had for forty years, he said. If they had, it likely wouldn't have made a difference. "I got one enjoyment in life and it's smoking," he said. "That's the only thing I do in life. I don't care. I got nobody to come home to. If it's going to kill me, I don't give a shit. I honestly don't give a shit."

The story of his life included becoming a parent while still a teenager himself, divorce, estrangement from his children, a workplace back injury, hearing loss from working on loud jobsites, and a suicide attempt. It started with a childhood lived in poverty in New Glasgow in northern Nova Scotia. "I grew up shithouse poor. I mean poor," he said, drawing out the "poor" to stress just how poor he meant. "I used to get off the school bus sometimes, change out of my school clothes into my hunting clothes, and if there wasn't a rabbit in one of my snares when I got home, back from my trip through the woods, there wasn't anything on that fucking table for dinner that night, buddy." There were four kids in the family and he was working on a farm baling hay by the time he was fourteen. Pelerine wasn't blaming anyone for how his life had turned out, describing it as a long run of bad luck, but he observed, "My life was fucked before it started." It's true that many people make choices that they know are bad for their health. It's also true that everyone comes from somewhere.

That social conditions contribute a great deal to whether people are healthy or sick has at times in the last forty years captured strong interest from senior levels of government. With support for the concept being voiced again in recent years, it's worth looking back at what happened previously, when the issue was at the top of the federal government's agenda. Action did not tend to match the rhetoric.

The seminal example in Canada came with a report written for then national health and welfare minister Marc Lalonde in 1974. Lalonde served in a cabinet that Prime Minister Pierre Trudeau headed. Titled *A New Perspective on the Health of Canadians*, Lalonde's report described a "health field" that was far broader than the health care system. In his preface to the report, Lalonde wrote that Canada's system of delivering health care to individuals was as good as any in the world. "The health care system, however, is only one of many ways of maintaining and improving health," he wrote. "Of equal or greater importance in increasing the number of illness-free days in the lives of Canadians have been the raising of the general standard of living, important sanitary measures for protecting public health, and advances in medical science."

The health of Canadians was under threat from what he identified as "the dark side of economic progress." He included "environmental pollution, city living, habits of indolence, the abuse of alcohol, tobacco and drugs, and eating patterns which put the pleasing of the senses above the needs of the human body." There was little being done to prevent those harms, Lalonde said. "For these environmental and behavioural threats to health, the organized health care system can do little more than serve as a catchment net for the victims."[7]

Lalonde acknowledged it would be a challenge to get people who were not sick to change their behaviours, and he saw a role for government leadership:

> The Government of Canada now intends to give to human biology, the environment and lifestyle as much attention as it has to the financing of the health care organization so that all four avenues to improved health are pursued with equal vigour. Its goal will continue to be not only to add years to our life but life to our years, so that all can enjoy the opportunities offered by increased economic and social justice.

He called for the provinces to work with the federal government on the new approach, and noted the concept had been endorsed by the provincial health ministers. He wrote:

> There are national health problems which know no provincial boundaries and which arise from causes imbedded in the social fabric of the nation as a whole. These problems cannot be solved solely by providing health services but rather must be attacked by offering the Canadian people protection, information and services through which they will themselves become partners with health professionals in the preservation and enhancement of their vitality.

Among the environmental conditions the report identified as contributing to poor health was income. "The number of economically deprived Canadians is still high, resulting in a lack of adequate housing and insufficient or inadequate clothing," said the report, published more than four decades ago. In another observation that remains relevant, the report identified an underlying philosophical shift that was happening in the country's attitude that had health consequences: "When a society increasingly pursues private pleasure by sacrificing its obligations to the common good, it invites stresses whose effect on health can be disastrous."

Lalonde championed the wider approach to health not only as the right thing to do, but as a practical way to restrain the escalating cost of the public health care system. The cost of providing health care in 1971 was $306.11 per person in Canada, most of which was for services provided to patients by doctors, nurses, dentists, pharmacists, hospitals and other providers. The report said it was "a substantial sum by any measure" and was prescient on the direction spending was headed: "The annual rate of cost escalation has been between 12% and 16%, which is far in excess of the economic growth of the country; if unchecked, health care costs will soon be beyond the capacity of society to finance them." In 2016, according to the Canadian Institute for Health Information, per person spending on health care was expected to reach $6,299.[8]

The innovative Canadian idea for health reform was noticed and picked up elsewhere. In a 1985 article in the *Canadian Journal of Public Health*, physician and public health advocate Trevor Hancock noted the Lalonde report's themes had been followed with similar reports in Britain, Sweden, the United States and elsewhere. The World Health Organization was supportive of the move away from dependence upon the biomedical model, he said, and quoted from the WHO's 1977 strategy for reaching its "Health for All by the Year 2000" goal:

Health does not exist in isolation. It is influenced by a complex
of environmental, social and economic factors ultimately related
to each other ... action undertaken outside the health sector can
have health effects much greater than those obtained within it.

Hancock argued that instead of just pursuing "public health policy" concerned with looking after the sick, governments should adopt "healthy public policy" that takes a broad approach. "Healthy public policy begins by questioning the givens: Why do we have to structure our society in such a way as to create ill health? Is there a way to structure our society so as to create health?" Healthy public policy would be more holistic and would deal, he wrote, "both with the health problems of the individual and the great global issues of the day—such as energy, food production, pollution and unemployment—that influence the health of humankind within the socio-environmental ecosystem of which we are a part."[9]

Now a public health professor at the University of Victoria, Hancock has described the need to look beyond an individual's immediate cause of death to find the causes of the causes and even the "causes of the causes of the causes."[10] An individual woman's death might be attributed to a stroke, but that's unlikely to be the full story. Maybe she had high blood pressure that was not detected or poorly controlled, Hancock wrote, "perhaps because she is a woman and lived in a rural or low-income community or on a reserve, where health care is less accessible. Or perhaps she could not afford the medication." It's worth asking why the person had high blood pressure in the first place, he continued. "A genetic predisposition? Obesity? A high-salt diet? Canadian diets are much too salty, and the Canadian food industry has resisted efforts to regulate salt content. A stressful life and work situation? Some combination of all these, and more?" With that broader perspective, many factors could take the blame for the death.

Despite the international interest, in Canada the Lalonde report led to little if any change. Writing a couple of decades after the report's release, Yale University political scientist Theodore Marmor and University of British Columbia economists Morris Barer and Robert Evans said that the report's good intentions and broad perspective were never really put into action. While the report's words sounded good, they wrote, "In practice, however, the breadth of policy response did not match the breadth of the 'new perspective' rhetoric. The role of 'life-styles' was seized upon with a vengeance, for a variety of different reasons, by politicians, health promoters, and the mass media."[11] The potentially revolutionary understanding that people make their choices within a wider context, and that they shouldn't really be understood as choices at all, was ignored. The authors wrote:

> The health promoters thus individualized both the root of the problem and many of the remedies. In this way they avoided challenging either the conventional world of work, income distribution, and control over the environment, or the conventional medical establishment. It was politically much safer to exhort individuals to live better, often implicitly blaming them for their own illnesses.

They gave the example of the Participaction program, which for years used television advertisements and other means to exhort Canadians to be more physically active. "The consistent theme throughout was that self-improvement constituted the key to a longer and healthier life. There was no suggestion, in any of these programs, that individual behaviour arose in and was shaped by a social and economic context, and that there might be some collective responsibility for changing that context."

Despite the lack of action, the sunny river of rhetoric kept flowing. A dozen years after the Lalonde report, Jake Epp built on its messages as the minister of national health and welfare in Prime Minister Brian Mulroney's government. He identified in his 1986 report three major challenges that the health system and policy of the day were failing to adequately address:

- disadvantaged groups have significantly lower life expectancy, poorer health and a higher prevalence of disability than the average Canadian;
- various forms of preventable diseases and injuries continue to undermine the health and quality of life of many Canadians;
- many thousands of Canadians suffer from chronic disease, disability, or various forms of emotional stress, and lack adequate community support to help them cope and live meaningful, productive and dignified lives.

"The times in which we live are characterized by rapid and irreversible social change," Epp wrote three decades ago. "Shifting family structures, an aging population and wider participation by women in the paid work force are all exacerbating certain health problems and creating pressure for new kinds of social support. They are forcing us also to seek new approaches for dealing effectively with the health concerns of the future." He proposed taking a "health promotion" approach that would complement the health care system.

Epp's idea was not, however, to simply nag Canadians better. The first challenge, his report said, would be finding ways to reduce the health inequities related to income in the country. "There is disturbing evidence which shows that despite Canada's superior health services system, people's health remains directly related to their economic status," he wrote, noting that people with low incomes lived shorter lives than those who made more money. "With respect to disabilities, the evidence is even more startling. Men in upper income groups can expect 14 more disability-free years than men with a low income; in the case of women, the difference is eight years." The causes for the differences were many, Epp said:

> Among low-income groups, people are more likely to die as a result of accidental falls, chronic respiratory disease, pneumonia, tuberculosis and cirrhosis of the liver. Also, certain conditions are more prevalent among Canadians in low-income groups; they include mental health disorders, high blood pressure and disorders of the joints and limbs.

The chances of experiencing health problems were greatest for people with low incomes who were older, unemployed, receiving welfare, single moms, Indigenous or immigrants.

Epp recognized that prompting people to change their behaviours was complex. "The realization that smoking, alcohol consumption and high-fat diets were contributing variously to lung cancer, cirrhosis of the liver, cardiovascular disease and motor vehicle accidents, led us to turn our attention to reducing risk behaviour and trying to change people's lifestyles," he wrote. There were reasons the approach had limited success, he said:

Unfortunately, the causal relationships between behaviour and health are not nearly as clear-cut as they are between "germs" and disease. Today's illnesses and injuries and the disabilities to which they give rise are the result of numerous interacting factors. This means that prevention is a far more complex undertaking than we may at one time have imagined.

Epp stressed that a focus on prevention didn't mean blaming people when they got sick or disabled, conditions that are "the outcome of wider social and economic circumstances." Blaming the individual was "based on the unrealistic notion that the individual has ultimate and complete control over life and death."

As well, there was a challenge Epp recognized with helping people cope with chronic conditions and mental health problems. "Obviously, we cannot afford to diminish our efforts to assist those who are suffering from serious mental illness; however, it is essential that we assign equal priority to helping people remain mentally healthy." The stress of modern life and changing social environment was difficult for many, especially women and people who were unemployed, Epp's report said. "We know that anxiety, tension, sadness, loneliness, insomnia and fatigue are often symptoms of mental stress which find expression in many forms, including child abuse, family violence, drug and alcohol misuse and suicide."[12]

Despite the enlightened perspective, all was not fixed by the time the Progressive Conservatives handed power back to the Liberals. And so the themes were repeated in a 1990s report the National Forum on Health prepared for Prime Minister Jean Chrétien and Health Minister David Dingwall. *Canada Health Action: Building on the Legacy* focused on sustaining the health care system, but also dedicated a section to building on the Lalonde and Epp reports. "We have known for some time that the better off people are in terms of income, social status, social networks, sense of control over their lives, self-esteem and education, the healthier they are likely to be," the report said. "We know that there is a gradient in health status, with health improving at each step up the slope of income, education and social status. We are all affected." It continued, "We are particularly concerned about the impact of poverty, unemployment, and cuts in social supports on the health of individuals, groups and communities." The effects of deprivation in childhood, which impairs brain development, can only partially be offset by later interventions, it said. "Government does set economic and social policies that have important consequences for the health of individuals and populations. A better balance must be struck between short-term economic imperatives and the long-term health and well-being of Canadians."[13]

Instead of putting the words into action, starting in 1995 Chrétien's government slashed transfer payments to the provinces for health, social services and education in an effort to reduce the federal debt. As Andrew Jackson, the national director of social and economic policy for the Canadian Labour Congress, wrote, "Putting the burden of debt reduction on social spending cuts rather than on taxation meant that the burden of Canadian deficit reduction fell on the lower end of the income distribution, and this was a significant factor behind the pronounced increase in Canadian income inequality over the 1990s." That had consequences, Jackson wrote. "The key lessons are that deep fiscal restraint is hugely damaging to the well-being of working families, and that better alternatives exist."[14]

Essentially, the federal government under both major parties has known for decades that poor health is closely tied to social inequity. And yet it has overseen widening inequality in Canada and in many cases has taken policy choices that have made matters worse.

The role of broader social policy in creating the conditions for people to be healthy has in recent decades been on the agenda in the United States as well. In 1992, when George H.W. Bush was president, the US Department of Health and Human Services released its *Healthy People 2000* report. The department's then secretary Louis W. Sullivan, a doctor, wrote in the foreword:

> The correlation between poor health and lower socio-economic status has been well documented, but that does not make it right or inevitable. Good health should not be seen, or, for that matter, be permitted to exist in fact, as a benefit for only those who can afford it; it should be available and accessible to every citizen.

Greater funding for the health care system could be expected to have little effect on many pressing conditions, wrote Sullivan:

> Medical care, alone, will not eliminate the devastating impact of chronic disease on the disadvantaged, nor will it reduce, as much as we would like, the rate of infant mortality or the burden of homicide and violence or any of the other "health" problems that are borne by the poor in our society.

Tellingly, he described the challenge as largely revolving around changing the behaviours and thinking of people who were vulnerable:

> If we are to extend the benefits of good health to all our people, it is crucial that we build in our most vulnerable populations what I have called a "culture of character," which is to say a culture, or a way of thinking and being, that actively promote responsible behavior and the adoption of lifestyles that are maximally conducive to good health. This is "prevention" in the broadest sense. It is also an absolute necessity, both because we are a humane and caring society and because, if we are to remain a vital society, we cannot afford to waste human resources. Good health must be an equal opportunity, available to all Americans.

Sullivan totalled up the amount the health care system spent each year on largely preventable diseases such as AIDS and including those caused by smoking, alcohol and drug use. "We would be terribly remiss if we did not seize the opportunity presented by health promotion and disease prevention to dramatically cut health-care costs, to prevent the premature onset of disease and disability, and to help all Americans achieve healthier, more productive lives," he concluded.[15]

The report itself laid out ways that families, communities, health professionals, the media and the government could help individuals make healthier choices, but failed to significantly address ways to reduce poverty. The closest it came was in a section on people with low income, where it observed that "improvements in education, job training, and other social services are necessary to erase the health effects of current income disparities." These were, however, out of the realm of public health, it claimed. As the report put it, "The leverage available to effect improvements is limited largely to the availability and the quality of health services."

The report bravely set targets in twenty-two areas, starting with "reduce overweight to a prevalence of no more than 20 percent among people aged 20 and older" by the year 2000. That would have been a 6 percent reduction from the report's 1976–80 baseline. The country has, of course, so far lost that battle. According to the National Center for Health Statistics at the Centers for Disease Control and Prevention, by 2013–14 the percentage of Americans who had a body mass index indicating they were overweight had reached 70.7 percent, or 3.5 times the goal, and a rising number were obese.[16]

The authors of the 1992 report also hoped to reduce the number of deaths from coronary heart disease from the 135 per 100,000 in 1987 to no more than 100. Heart disease is closely related to smoking, alcohol use, blood pressure, diabetes, stress and other factors linked to how people live. It too went the other way. In 2014, the most recent data available as of this writing, the disease remained the number one killer of Americans, taking the lives of 614,348 people that year. That's a rate of 192.7 deaths from the disease per 100,000 people, or about 50 percent higher than the 1987 baseline and 90 percent more than the target. The rate of deaths from strokes had also risen, and was double the target set in the report. The morbidity rate from cancer, the second leading cause of death in 2014, was up more than 40 percent. The rate of suicide deaths had grown too.

Whatever the United States had done since the 1992 report, as a country it had become significantly sicker. The failure speaks to widespread misery, early deaths and a monstrous waste of potential that could well have been avoided.

In Canada in the years since the vision of the Lalonde and Epp reports, gains had been elusive as well. In a 2015 report, the Canadian Institute for Health Information found that despite heavy spending on health care there was still a persistent health outcome divide between rich and poor.

"Over the past decade, little or no progress has been made in reducing inequalities in health by income level in Canada," it said. Specifically:

> Since the early 2000s, inequalities have widened for [three] of the 16 health indicators that were studied and did not change for 11 of them. While inequalities did narrow for the remaining [two] indicators, this was the result of an undesirable "levelling down" effect — in other words, health worsened among the richest Canadians while at the same time there was no change among the lowest income group.

For example, in all but the highest income group, people were rating their mental health lower than they had in 2003. Infant mortality continued to be tied to income as well, the report said. "If all families had experienced the same low rates of infant deaths as those in the highest income group, there would have been 300 fewer deaths in 2011." Obesity continued to grow in every province and at all income levels, but with continued gaps between rich and poor, particularly for women. "Women in lower-income households continue to have a prevalence of obesity that is 1.5 times higher than that among women in higher-income households (20% versus 13%)," the CIHI report said.[17]

While most Canadians had reduced smoking since 2003, there was no change in the rate among the 40 percent of adults in the bottom two income levels. Among people under seventy-five years old, those in the highest income group were less likely to be hospitalized with chronic obstructive pulmonary disease than they had been in 2001, but the rate of hospitalizations had risen for lower-income Canadians. Smoking is the leading cause of chronic obstructive pulmonary disease and both smoking and hospitalization for COPD are more prevalent among people who are poorer. According to the CIHI, "the smoking rate is almost twice as high for the lowest-income Canadians as for the highest-income Canadians, and the COPD hospitalization rate is more than [three] times as high for the lowest-income Canadians compared with the highest-income group."

Put another way, not only are poorer people more likely to smoke, they are more likely to get sick from it. It's a phenomenon that epidemiologist

Michael Marmot and physician Fraser Mustard described this way a couple decades ago: "Those few men in the higher grades who smoked were at lower risk *from smoking-related diseases* than were smokers in the lower grades, though at each grade (with the exception of the bottom grade), smokers were at higher risk than nonsmokers. Smoking does kill; but it is clearly not the main explanation for the social gradient in mortality."[18]

According to the CIHI report, hospitalization for COPD is generally considered avoidable, and those who receive effective chronic disease management and primary care have a better hope of staying out of the hospital, which is where savings are to be had. On average, a hospitalization for COPD costs $8,000, it said. "If all Canadians experienced the same low rates of hospitalization for COPD as the highest income earners, there would be more than 18,000 fewer hospitalizations, which translates into $150 million in health sector savings annually."

Nor was Canada doing as well as it could providing help outside the health care system to people. The CIHI report argued that major progress on health inequities was unlikely without taking a broader social approach, including boosting people's incomes. "Income is not the sole factor that explains health inequalities, but it is a fundamentally important variable and is related to other important measures of socio-economic status such as education," the report said. Lower taxes and cuts to social assistance in the mid-1990s had contributed to a widening gap, it said.

The report suggested various ways to reduce income inequality, including increasing taxes and transfers, increasing minimum wages, acting on poverty reduction strategies and spending on education and training programs. "The experience of countries with reasonably well-developed social programs suggests that a combination of universal and targeted programs is necessary to address inequalities in health, since there is evidence of poorer health all along the income gradient and not just among the lowest-income earners."

In Canada, however, successive governments have short-changed those programs for years. Juha Mikkonen and Dennis Raphael at York University wrote in 2010 that Canadian governments were offering protections and supports that were well below what would be available in other industrialized, wealthy countries. They used figures from the Organisation for Economic Co-operation and Development comparing its thirty members:

> Canada ranks 24th of 30 countries and spends only 17.8 percent of gross domestic product (GDP) on public expenditures. Among OECD countries for which data is available, Canada is amongst the lowest public spenders on early childhood education and care (26th of 27), seniors' benefits and supports (26th of 29), social assistance payments (22nd of 29), unemployment benefits (23rd of 28), benefits and services for people with disabilities (27th of 29), and supports and benefits to families with children (25th of 29).

And when it came to work, arrangements in Canada tended to be more precarious than elsewhere in the OECD. "The OECD calculates an employment protection index of rules and regulations that protects employment and provides benefits to temporary workers. Canada performs very poorly on this index achieving a score that was ranked 26th of 28 nations."[19] Canada remained in that position in 2013, the most recent year for which rankings were available (see Figure 1.2).

Sociologist and former federal health minister Monique Bégin described the situation in Canada in the foreword to *Social Determinants of Health: The Canadian Facts*:

> The truth is that Canada—the ninth richest country in the world— is so wealthy that it manages to mask the reality of poverty, social exclusion and discrimination, the erosion of employment quality, its adverse mental health outcomes, and youth suicides. While one of the world's biggest spenders in health care, we have one of the worst records in providing an effective social safety net. What good does it do to treat people's illnesses, to then send them back to the conditions that made them sick?

Bégin, who was also a member of the WHO Commission on Social Determinants of Health, argued in the 2010 document that the political tide was changing in Canada, increasing the public interest in a more

Fig 1.2 Employment Protection, OECD Nations, 2013

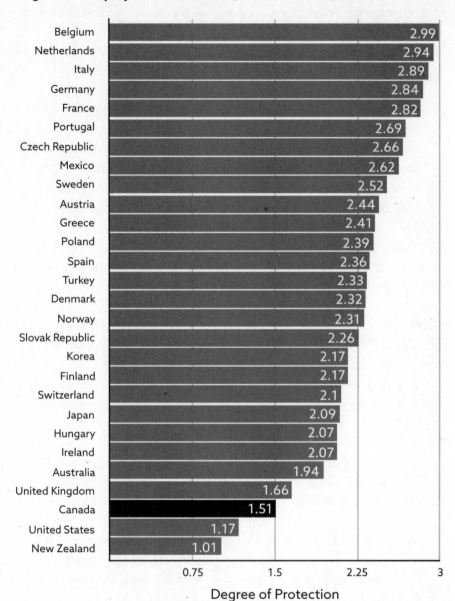

	Degree of Protection
Belgium	2.99
Netherlands	2.94
Italy	2.89
Germany	2.84
France	2.82
Portugal	2.69
Czech Republic	2.66
Mexico	2.62
Sweden	2.52
Austria	2.44
Greece	2.41
Poland	2.39
Spain	2.36
Turkey	2.33
Denmark	2.32
Norway	2.31
Slovak Republic	2.26
Korea	2.17
Finland	2.17
Switzerland	2.1
Japan	2.09
Hungary	2.07
Ireland	2.07
Australia	1.94
United Kingdom	1.66
Canada	1.51
United States	1.17
New Zealand	1.01

Degree of Protection

Source   OECD, *Strictness of Employment Protection*, 2013

collective approach. "Following years of a move towards the ideology of individualism, a growing number of Canadians are anxious to reconnect with the concept of a just society and the sense of solidarity it envisions. Health inequities are not a problem just of the poor. It is our challenge and it is about public policies and political choices and our commitments to making these happen."[20]

After the Liberals were elected in 2015 on a platform that promised increased social spending, it seemed likely that the broad approach to supporting a healthier population would be revived. Prime Minister Justin Trudeau made Jane Philpott, a doctor representing Markham-Stouffville in Ontario, the health minister. There's no question she came to the job with a better understanding than most health ministers about what it is that makes people healthy. In 2014, when her daughter Bethany was entering medical school at McMaster University in Hamilton, Philpott wrote a blog post offering thirty pieces of advice based on her own experiences as a doctor, which included nine years working in Niger. She wrote:

> Remember what really makes people sick and what makes them well. You will be taught about immunology, pathology, infections, and much more. But you already know that the social determinants of health actually set the stage for all those biomedical actors … Do your part to influence those social determinants. Speak up when you see the impact of poverty, unemployment, violence and more.[21]

You would think that as health minister, Philpott would have been ideally placed to act on that knowledge. But in his mandate letter to Philpott, who held the position for the first two years of the government's mandate, Trudeau emphasized her job supporting the health care system. "Your overarching goal will be to strengthen our publicly-funded universal health care system and ensure that it adapts to new challenges," the letter said. In doing so it gave priority to the system, not health.

Philpott was to work with provincial and territorial governments "to support them in their efforts to make home care more available, prescription drugs more affordable, and mental health care more accessible."

Mikkonen and Raphael listed 14 social determinants of health:

1. Income and Income Distribution
2. Education
3. Unemployment and Job Security
4. Employment and Working Conditions
5. Early Childhood Development
6. Food Insecurity
7. Housing
8. Social Exclusion
9. Social Safety Network
10. Health Services
11. Aboriginal Status
12. Gender
13. Race
14. Disability

As for public health, Trudeau wanted Philpott to increase vaccination rates, eliminate or reduce the amount of trans fat and salt in processed foods, restrict the advertising of unhealthy food and drinks to children, and improve food labelling. The words "social determinants of health" were unmentioned.[22]

In an interview in the summer of 2017, York University professor Raphael sounded discouraged by the signals out of Ottawa. "I don't see any evidence at all that anything's getting better," he said. "I'm not in a good mental space in terms of us moving this forward."

As we approached fifty years since the Lalonde report, the skepticism seemed justified. The need was as strong as ever to take a broad social approach to support people to be healthy, but there was little sign of progress. Public discussion about health continued to focus on the health care system, even as it struggled to respond to crises in mental health and addictions. Homelessness, a symptom of what was broken, was growing in many of our cities and too many children continued to grow up in poverty. Five decades of experience had demonstrated that knowledge was not enough for us to make better public policy choices.

CHAPTER 2

Diagnosis

Health Care and
Canadian Pride

My most extensive direct experience with the health care system was in 2001, the year my first daughter was born. My wife, Suzanne, gave birth to Annie in our home, where everything went well up until the delivery. Afterwards, however, Suzanne kept bleeding heavily despite the midwives making sure the entire placenta had come out, giving her shots of oxytocin and confirming her uterus had contracted. With Annie tucked in the crook of one arm, I dialled 9-1-1 with my free hand. When the ambulance arrived to take Suzanne to the hospital, the workers lifted her and she lost consciousness, and her head and shoulders slumped suddenly forward. Clutching our newborn to my chest, I climbed into a car driven by one of the midwives.

At the hospital, Suzanne's eyes were open but their whites had turned yellow. She was in a room buzzing with doctors and nurses. A nurse wanted to know if Suzanne had any allergies or if she was taking any drug or homeopathic substance that might have thinned her blood. An obstetrician ordered blood tests. Another doctor recommended blood transfusions, which were soon delivered. Suzanne was taken to the intensive care unit where she was given more blood products and hooked up to tubes delivering saline and antibiotics. A catheter was inserted. A tube through her nose allowed gas and muddy fluid to escape from her stomach. Outside there was a small "grief" room with armchairs and a box of tissues.

Altogether we were in the hospital for twelve days. Space was found for me and Annie on the mother and babe ward. Eventually Suzanne was diagnosed with HELLP syndrome, which stands for hemolysis, elevated liver enzymes and low platelets. Her liver and kidneys were in serious trouble and she didn't have enough platelets available for clotting after the birth. It's a rare condition with unknown causes. The only "cure" is to give birth and then hope for recovery. A doctor estimated Suzanne's chances of survival had been 50 percent. One of the nurses said it was closer to one out of five. She did survive, which she says has increased the gratitude she has for each day.

And the experience of course made us grateful for the health care system—the hospital, doctors and nurses. They saw us through a scary time without bankrupting us; in fact the only thing we paid for directly was the ambulance ride to the hospital. The figure sounds about right to me when Doctor Danielle Martin tells Americans, "In public polls, 94 per cent of Canadians say that our health-care system is a source of personal and collective pride—even more than ice hockey." I agree when she says, "Single-payer health care is a symbol to us of what it truly means to be Canadian: that we take care of each other."[1] Many of us love our health care system.

Despite that love, it has been a national pastime to fret about the state of Canadian health care. At the time of my daughter's birth, much of the rhetoric around the health care system was that it was in crisis and that more private care was needed. Stories of waiting lists and the system's occasional failures dominated. It was a storyline at times fed by people working in the system, their unions and supportive opposition parties. But the care we experienced in the hospital seemed to us to be thorough. There was a battery of specialists who continued to follow Suzanne even after we'd returned home. A social worker was available to talk with in the hospital. Later there were appointments with a counsellor to follow up. A public health nurse visited us at home and there was help with breastfeeding through a nearby clinic. Our experience was at odds with the stories about health care being in crisis.

As that daughter turned sixteen in 2017, the public discussion around health care continued to centre on a system suffering from underfunding. Stories of crowded hospitals, difficulties finding a family doctor, and long wait-lists, particularly for orthopaedic surgeries and MRI screenings, were common. Brian Day, a Vancouver doctor, was the public face of a long awaited BC Supreme Court challenge to sections of the Medicare Protection Act. The Cambie Surgeries Corporation was arguing that laws preventing patients from paying extra for speedier treatment violated their constitutional rights, which critics saw as an attempt to give better access to care to people who were willing to pay. The overall impression was of a system that was sick, but with cures being offered that could well make matters worse.

Adding to the unease, Canadian health care has failed to measure up well in some international comparisons. The Commonwealth Fund, a group in the United States that compares health care in eleven developed countries, in its 2017 report ranked Canada's system in ninth place overall, which was a step up from its report released three years earlier (see Figure 2.1). The United States held the bottom spot, spending far more than any of the other countries—fully 16.6 percent of its gross domestic product—to achieve worse results. While Canada was in the middle for "care process and administrative efficiencies," the country lagged on access, equity and health care outcomes.

The "access" measure, where Canada did worse than every country in the study except the US, included affordability and timeliness, covering both problems paying for dental or other care and waiting times for elective or non-emergency surgery. Canada received low scores for people not having after-hours access to care without going to an emergency room, waiting more than two hours for care in emergency, not being able to see a nurse or doctor on the same or next day when seeking care and long wait times to see a specialist or get some kinds of surgery.

As for equity, in the United Kingdom, the Netherlands and Sweden, the Commonwealth Fund found, "there are relatively small differences between lower- and higher-income adults on the 11 measures related to timeliness, financial barriers to care, and patient-centered care." Canada, along with the US and France, had larger disparities related to how much money people make and the care they receive. "These were especially large on measures related to financial barriers, such as skipping needed doctor visits or dental care, forgoing treatments or tests, and not filling prescriptions because of the cost," the report said. In the US, high infant

Fig 2.1 **Health Care System Performance Compared to Spending**

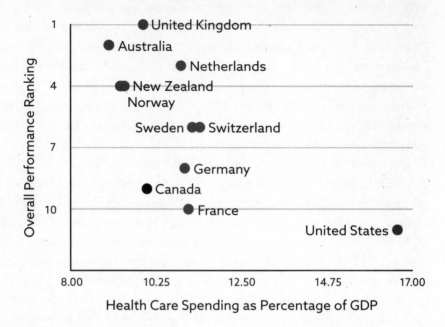

Source Commonwealth Fund, with data from the OECD for the year 2014

mortality and low life expectancy showed a need for better preventative care. "The high level of inequity in the U.S. health care system intensifies the problem. For the first time in decades, midlife mortality for less-educated Americans is rapidly increasing." In other words, a long-term trend had reversed and some groups of Americans were beginning to die younger. Canada was doing better, but not much.[2]

It can be difficult to get a sense of the overall state of health care, to figure out what's anecdotal, what's needless worry, and what's a real problem. Emily Nicholas Angl, a Torontonian who is a speaker and advisor for Patients Canada and who works with Dr. Mike Evans promoting public health, said in an interview in 2015 that from a patient's point of view the system can appear fractured and disjointed. "There almost is no big picture to have," she said. The delivery of health care in

Canada, and the experience of patients and their families, depends not just on provincial and territorial governments, but on local hospitals and medical offices, she said. As a patient who over the course of ten years had extensive care for various conditions, thirty-three-year-old Angl said, "I had a positive experience in terms of the people, but in terms of the actual system, it felt like my job." Which is to say it took a lot of work at her end to navigate her care, a problem for people in need of help. "I think it doesn't feel very much like a system," Angl said. "It feels like a lot of different institutions that are quite siloed …. It's very much small pockets of health systems."

The local differences and the need to self-advocate for care lead to inequities in a system that is supposed to be universal. "There is want for some sort of consistency or direction for making things better across Canada," Angl said, pointing out that leadership needed to come from the federal government. Issues like a national pharmacare program, doctor-assisted dying, integrating services and creating electronic health records would all benefit from national leadership, Angl said.

It was a theme in line with an editorial that appeared in the *Canadian Medical Association Journal* (*CMAJ*) ahead of the 2015 election and was critical of what it described as the government's dereliction of health planning. The journal's deputy editor, Matthew Stanbrook, a doctor who also teaches at the Institute of Health Policy, Management and Evaluation at the University of Toronto, argued that the federal government appeared to be trying to get out of health care. "For much of the last decade, Canadian federal health policy has been conspicuous by its absence," he wrote. "Many essential aspects of health care are a federal responsibility, and our biggest, most complex problems in the health care system cannot be solved without federal leadership. Without such leadership, Canadians will continue to suffer." One necessary priority was making access to pharmaceuticals more affordable, he wrote. "Lack of universal drug insurance places at risk the lives and health of far too many Canadians who cannot afford the increasingly expensive medications they need," he said, noting a national plan would cost little and provide great benefit to many people.[3]

The need for a national drug plan was at the top of the list for Michael Decter, a former Ontario deputy minister of health and financial advisor who chairs the board of Patients Canada. There were two "real embarrassments" in Canadian health care, he said. The first was that half a million people in Atlantic Canada had no drug coverage whatsoever. "That's pretty glaring," he said, noting that in that region stories of communities helping neighbours raise money to buy expensive drug treatments are common. The other fundamental problem, Decter said, was the "abysmal" life expectancy and health status of First Nations, Inuit and Métis people in the country, attributable mainly to the social determinants of health.

Decter said despite fundamental problems, he felt health care was less under threat in 2015 than it had been in the late 1990s. The increased budget since 2006 with transfers rising by 6 percent a year had helped, he said, though much of the increase had gone to providers rather than spurring a shift from a system centred around doctors and hospitals to one that's more community based. As provinces faced making do with smaller increases after 2017, funding was needed to help find innovative ways to deliver care, he said. Many people aren't getting care they need when and where they need it. "There's a lot to be improved in the system."

Despite regional variations, across the country hospitals faced some common problems, said the Canadian Medical Association's past president, Chris Simpson. "Emergency rooms are kind of like the barometer of the system," said Simpson, a cardiologist based in Kingston. In travels throughout Canada he had found crowded emergency rooms from coast to coast. "Everywhere I went the story was the same," he said. Those problems are a symptom of a larger problem with Canadian health care, he said. "The main issue is this over reliance on hospitals and doctors to solve all our health care problems." The CMA was campaigning to improve care for seniors, which Simpson said would relieve the pressure on hospitals and emergency rooms. "We think if we can fix seniors care … we'll go a long way to fixing what's wrong with health care in general."

Building the system around doctors and hospitals may have made sense in the 1960s and '70s, but the population had since shifted, Simpson said. As the Canadian population aged, health practitioners were spending much more time helping people manage chronic conditions. "You don't need hospitals to do that, but that's where they're coming." These are people who could be looked after cheaper—and better—outside the hospital, he said, adding that a hospital bed costs the government $1,000 a day compared to $150 a day for a bed in a long-term care facility. "We fundamentally don't think there needs to be more money in the system," Simpson said. Health care takes up about 11 percent of Canada's GDP. "We don't need to spend more than that, but we need to spend very differently." There's an opportunity for the federal government to set national standards and bring the provinces together to help them provide better care than they could on their own, he said. The system can keep spinning its wheels and have differing levels of care across the country, or arrive at a national vision: "For me it's as simple as that."

The need for federal leadership was central in David Naylor's prescription for fixing Canadian health care as well. A physician and medical researcher who served as president of the University of Toronto until 2013, Naylor chaired an advisory panel on health care innovation whose report came out shortly before the 2015 election. After a year of consultation, discussion and reflection, the panel concluded that medicare was aging badly. "An overview of the OECD indicators on health care spending and performance suggests that, on a value-for-money basis, Canada is not where it should be," Naylor told me via email. The Commonwealth Fund's assessment of Canadian health care should also give people pause, he said:

> The weaknesses crop up in different ways. Poor integration of services, leading to problems with continuity of care and sharing of information. Continued challenges with waiting times for a range of specialist services. A low proportion of Canadians who can see their family doctor within 24 hours as compared to sister nations. Underuse of health information technology and virtual care. And a lack of coverage of services for a wide range of professionals other than physicians. We're also just about the only country with universal health care that doesn't also have universal coverage for prescribed pharmaceuticals.

That lack of integration across "service silos in each province and territory" has led to the underdevelopment of information systems that can operate with each other across borders, he said, which has been "a barrier to innovation in all aspects of health care."

Meanwhile our drug spending is high, in part because of high prices, but also because of the number of prescriptions being written and the drugs that doctors choose to prescribe, Naylor said. "If a new drug saves costs elsewhere in the system, or has broader economic benefits by keeping people healthier and more productive, those considerations are not always fairly reflected in decisions about its adoption," he said. "Thus, we not only need to get tough on prices and procurement. We also need to align incentives in support of prudent prescribing, including faster uptake of those new drugs that actually add value to the system." To help lower-income and older Canadians deal with growing out-of-pocket expenses, the panel suggested introducing a refundable health tax credit. "As we said in the report, the tax credit approach is partly about buying time until we figure out how to modernize medicare," Naylor said. "But realistically, there will always be some services that are not covered by the public purse."

There are some areas where Canada does well. "Our system has notable strengths, starting with an absence of financial barriers for medical and hospital services," Naylor said. "We also have low administrative costs, capable managers, and thousands of outstanding health professionals." But pride in Canadian health care was blocking making it better. "Canadians are often distracted by self-congratulatory comparisons with the expensive chaos in health care south of the border," he said. "What we could have done instead was to cherry-pick the best ideas from the non-profit health care sector in the US. If we had reached across the border, and borrowed integrated delivery systems and bundled funding for a wide range of our services, Canada would be still a world leader in universal health care today."

Naylor said he could understand why successive Canadian federal governments, which help fund but don't directly deliver most health care in the country, had been reluctant to be more involved in setting the direction for provinces and territories. The federal government could impose conditions on health care transfers, as the CMAJ and others had called for, but had mostly chosen not to in recent years. Naylor said:

> In effect, Ottawa gets blamed for problems in health care but doesn't have constitutional authority to make changes. The reality, however, is that Conservative and Liberal governments in Ottawa created medicare in three key legislative steps: Cost-sharing for universal hospitalization insurance in the 1950s; cost-sharing for medical services insurance in the 1960s; and consolidation of cost-sharing conditions under the Canada Health Act of 1984. Canada is still one country, and the world looks at medicare as a national program. Like it or not, Ottawa can't simply throw money over the wall and walk away.

Asked to what degree more money should be seen as the cure, Naylor said it's hard to insist that transfer payments to the provinces should compound at 6 percent annually when the economy is growing much slower than that. At the same time, he added, some of the smaller provinces would have a hard time managing the impact of an aging population on their finances and on their health and social programs. "Health care has always been a political minefield, in Canada and elsewhere," Naylor said. "People all over the planet put a huge premium on their health. That means doctors and nurses in particular are tough political opponents. They are linked to something essential to everyone. They interact with millions of Canadians each year. And they are credible in ways that politicians will never be." Making the needed changes would require officials to put the public interest ahead of short-term political goals, he concluded. "Above all, we have a worrisome deficit of long-term thinking in business and government alike."

During the 2015 election campaign there was little discussion about health policy, despite attempts by organizations including the Canadian Medical Association and the union Unifor to put it at the top of the agenda. What debate there was mostly centred around the Conservative government's decision to limit the increase in transfers to the provinces for health care. Instead of continuing to rise by 6 percent a year, the transfers would be linked to growth in the economy, with a minimum annual increase of 3 percent.

The commitments on health from the eventual winners, Justin Trudeau and the Liberal Party, revolved around working more closely with the provinces. In a letter to the premiers, Trudeau wrote:

> If my party forms government, we will call a federal-provincial meeting to reach a long-term agreement on health care funding. A Liberal government will reengage in areas where there is direct federal responsibility, including health promotion, support to caregivers, and First Nations' health, and will meet with the Premiers to talk about how to strengthen health care.

Hedy Fry, who had represented Vancouver Centre as a Liberal since 1993 and served as her party's health critic, is a physician and former president of the BC Medical Association. "If nothing is done about health care it will hit a critical point very soon," she told me, citing Canada's drop over the years in the Commonwealth Fund's assessment. "It's a race to the bottom for us." Long-term care is a focus for the Liberals, Fry said, adding there needs to be a shift to more care in the community and acute care in a hospital should only be for when it is medically needed.

As for a national pharmacare program, Fry said the then Liberal government in 2004 addressed pharmacare in health accord commitments that Stephen Harper's Conservative government later abandoned. "We understand the issue," she said. Rather than commit to a national program, she said, "We want to present it to the provinces and have a discussion and negotiation." Fry also pointed out that research out of UBC showed a pharmacare program could pay for itself. She made a comparison to other wealthy countries in the Organisation for Economic Co-operation and Development. "We pay more for drugs per capita than any other developed country in the OECD. We need to fix that."

Once the Liberals formed government, they faced continuing pressure to increase spending on health care. In December 2016, as Prime Minister Trudeau and the country's premiers prepared to meet, the Canadian Health Coalition released a statement saying, "In order to ensure health care is able to meet the needs of a growing and aging

Canadian population, the Prime Minister must be willing to put more money on the table and the premiers must be willing to accept it with strings attached to health care spending." It quoted national coordinator Adrienne Silnicki opposing tying health funding to economic growth. "No one has been talking about how to ensure the funding can continue to deliver the services Canadians need ... We need funding that reflects the needs of Canadians, not the fluctuations of markets." The coalition cited a report from Ontario's Financial Accountability Office that found it would require a 5.2 percent budget increase just to maintain the existing level of health services. It called for increased spending tied to a seniors care plan and national public drug plan.[4]

And in July 2017, when Trudeau and the premiers were meeting in Edmonton, the Canadian Health Coalition put out another statement quoting Silnicki:

> In the 2015 election, the Trudeau Government promised to provide collaborative federal leadership while negotiating a new Health Accord with provinces and territories ... But instead the Federal Government split apart the provinces and territories and made bilateral agreements that will amount to a $33 billion cut over 10 years. The bilateral deals ignore the need to create national pharmacare, take action on a national seniors strategy, and do a better job enforcing the Canada Health Act to stop unlawful billing by private clinics.[5]

The coalition describes itself as "a public advocacy organization dedicated to the protection and improvement of Medicare." At least ten of the seventeen members of the CHC's executive and board in 2017 came directly from the labour movement and the chair of the board was Pauline Worsfold, from the Canadian Federation of Nurses Unions.[6]

The federal New Democratic Party has also pressed for increased spending on the health care system. In the fall of 2016 the party announced it was making the preservation of public health care its number one priority. Don Davies, the NDP's health critic, was quoted saying, "I think Canadians may not be aware of the serious threats that confront medicare ... We've got to strongly be on the Liberal government's case to make sure that they actually increase funding, and make sure that the federal government is increasing resources to the provinces."[7]

The government, however, resisted pressure to pour more money into the system. They negotiated hard with the provinces to restrict the increases to health transfer payments to 3 percent plus inflation and tied the increased money to particular areas, including improving mental health care and addiction treatment. The decision will leave some needs unmet, as the critics point out. However there is a strong case, as Naylor and others made, that the government doesn't need to spend more money to improve the health of Canadians. But it does need to spend better.

CHAPTER 3

Bad Habits

Wasteful Spending and Ignored Needs

No question there are gaps in the health care available to Canadians. There's clearly a need for a national drug plan, which would help make prescriptions more affordable and provide an opportunity for a centralized body to decide which drugs are worth paying for and which are not. Mental health care needs to be more readily available. Too many people, particularly among the vulnerable sections of the population, suffer with illnesses that are preventable or that could have been mitigated with earlier treatment. And it makes little sense that dentistry, particularly for children, isn't included in Canada's universal system, which offers care for the whole body but leaves out the mouth. Then there are the needs outside the health care system, the broader contributors to health that the Lalonde report identified more than forty years ago and which remain unaddressed. Some of the measures have the potential to save money, but others will require new spending. If the system is already stretched, where is the needed funding to come from?

A good place to start would be with a careful examination of where health dollars are spent now. While there are gaps in what's offered, paradoxically, many observers have pointed out there are also times in Canada when too much care is provided. Any money that's routinely wasted could be redirected to needs that aren't being met, or to measures outside the health care system with the potential to make Canadians healthier overall.

Wendy Levinson, a professor of medicine at the University of Toronto, has been a leading critic of waste in health care. She has written that Canadians get at least one million unnecessary medical tests, treatments and procedures every year. The figure comes from the Canadian Institute for Health Information, which released the research in partnership with Choosing Wisely Canada, an organization Levinson founded. Unnecessary tests can lead to people receiving care they don't need, she said, which exposes them to potential harm. "Unnecessary care could be a prescription drug, a diagnostic test or a medical procedure that doesn't improve a patient's health outcomes and isn't backed by the best available evidence. It may also involve risks and harmful side-effects." Besides potentially doing harm, she said, such care strains the resources of the health care system.[1]

Even giving birth, which is the most common reason for women to be hospitalized, can lead to unnecessary care, Levinson has said. There were 350,000 babies born in Canadian hospitals in 2016, nearly a third of them by caesarean-section delivery.[2] Was every one of those surgeries necessary? Probably not, considering the Canadian rate is high, more than double the World Health Organization's suggestion that ideally, no more than about 15 percent of births should be by caesarean. As the WHO website explained, "New studies reveal that when caesarean section rates rise towards 10% across a population, the number of maternal and newborn deaths decreases. But when the rate goes above 10%, there is no evidence that mortality rates improve." The WHO also issued a statement in 2015 saying that while unnecessary caesarean sections could pull resources away from other parts of a health care system, decisions should be made on a case-by-case basis, rather than with target rates in mind.[3]

Midwives talk about the "cascade of interventions" where one unnecessary test leads to further unnecessary interventions that may not lead to better outcomes for mother or baby. Episiotomies—making a cut in the moments ahead of delivery to widen the vaginal opening in an attempt to reduce tearing—are still done routinely, although as Levinson and Saskatchewan doctor George Carson point out, "evidence now shows this pre-emptive cut can lead to increased pain, longer periods of healing and potential complications down the road." They conclude,

"Sometimes, in an emergency, an episiotomy is needed but it should not be done routinely."[4]

There are many reasons a person might get care they don't really need. Levinson has been quoted saying patients contribute by demanding cutting-edge tests and treatments they've read about on the internet, and that some doctors may choose to appease those patients, perhaps in hopes of protecting themselves from a lawsuit if something is missed.[5] A patient may feel reassured to receive a particular test or treatment, and there are plenty of stories of having to advocate for care that really is needed. And doctors who give unneeded care doubtless believe they are acting in the patient's best interest. But as Levinson pointed out, many routine tests are done automatically in the health care system, including by doctors who may order a procedure out of habit, even if more recent evidence proves it will have little or no benefit.

My friend Alan Cassels, an author and health policy researcher, has made a career illustrating the point that sometimes the care we pay for doesn't work, or can even lead to harm. His 2012 book *Seeking Sickness: Medical Screening and the Misguided Hunt for Disease* considers the evidence on various kinds of tests, including whole body scans, mammograms and genetic screening.[6] Over lunch one day he showed me an infographic about the benefits and harms of the prostate specific antigen, or PSA, test for prostate cancer. Out of 1,000 men who get screened, there will be as many as 120 who do not have prostate cancer, but test positive anyway. They'll experience some anxiety and undergo a biopsy, a procedure that comes with a risk of infection, pain and bleeding. Another 110 will be diagnosed with prostate cancer and will likely feel grateful for treatment, even if they are among the 50 who experience complications that include infections, sexual dysfunction and bladder or bowel control problems. Four or five of them will die. That is, by the way, pretty much exactly the same number of deaths as there would have been in a group of 1,000 men who never got screened. The money spent on screening 1,000 men—with all the associated anxiety, pain and side effects—prevents somewhere between one and zero deaths.[7]

According to the Canadian Cancer Society, men need to discuss the benefits and the risks of the PSA test with their doctors. Finding prostate cancer early, before it grows large or spreads beyond the prostate, can mean treatment will be more successful, its website says. At the same time, there are risks, starting with the fact that about 75 percent of the men who test positive will not actually have prostate cancer. "A false-positive result can lead to unnecessary follow-up testing that is more invasive, such as repeated biopsies. It can also cause men and their families unnecessary anxiety and distress."

Nor does a negative test necessarily mean a man doesn't have cancer. For about 15 percent of men who do have prostate cancer, the test won't show it, which the cancer society cautioned could lead to misplaced confidence, symptoms being ignored, and a decision to skip treatment that is in fact needed.

There is also a risk of diagnosing prostate cancer that is present but that would never pose a serious risk to a man's health, the website says. "Research shows that 23%–42% of prostate cancers that are found with PSA testing may never need to be treated," it explained. In many cases, prostate cancer is slow growing; it will be present when a man dies, but won't have caused his death. The thing is, the Canadian Cancer Society website points out, once a man has tested positive for prostate cancer, most often he will opt to have it treated regardless of whether or not that treatment is needed. "Unnecessary follow-up testing and treatment put a man at risk for problems, including erectile dysfunction and loss of bladder control," it says.[8] Despite the issues with the PSA test, in recent years there's been pressure on provincial governments to fund the test for all men, not just those considered at high risk for prostate cancer.

Other tests that are frequently given in situations where they aren't warranted are CT scans, according to the CIHI and Choosing Wisely study mentioned earlier. In the years the study covered, CT scans, X-rays that produce a cross-section image of a body, were given to 30 percent of patients who went to an emergency department in Ontario or Alberta with a minor head injury. They are not without risk. As Levinson explained, "CT scans deliver strong X-ray radiation. Exposure to this radiation can increase lifetime cancer risk."[9] Instead of automatically ordering a scan, she recommended, all doctors should use a set of questions designed to allow them to assess the severity of the person's injury before deciding if the scan is really needed, thus sparing them from the unneeded and harmful exposure to radiation. Similarly, one out of ten seniors regularly use sleeping pills and other sedative hypnotics—which are only recommended for short-term use—even though they increase the risk of injuries from falls or car accidents.

In total the study looked at eight areas, including scans for lower back pain, mammography screening for younger women deemed at low risk for breast cancer, and the prescribing of atypical antipsychotics to children and youth. Among low-risk patients, as many as 30 percent were receiving medical tests they likely didn't need, the study found.[10] While there's a role for better policy and practices for those working in the system, patients can also ask the right questions to avoid unneeded care, Levinson wrote. She recommended asking: Do I really need this test, treatment or procedure? What are the downsides? Are there simpler, safer options? What happens if I do nothing?[11]

The CIHI and Choosing Wisely report didn't look at how much such waste costs, but the amount would be high. The *Journal of the American Medical Association* put the price of overtreatment at as much as $226 billion (USD) in 2011 in the United States.[12] A similar report from the Institute of Medicine in the United States in 2012 looked more broadly at medical waste and found that $750 billion (USD) may be spent needlessly each year in that country, the bulk of it on procedures that were unneeded.[13]

The Dartmouth Atlas of Health Care, a long-term study done at a research institute at Dartmouth College in New Hampshire, is frequently cited as the source of the finding that as much as 30 percent of health care spending in the United States is unnecessary. The finding was based on the observation that some regions spent more than others without getting better results. If all regions could safely reduce their spending to match the low-spending areas without sacrificing quality, there would be large savings, they found. And since even the low-cost regions could likely find savings, 30 percent overspending is likely an underestimate, the institute's website said. The issue largely has to do with what receives money, it said:

> Dartmouth research comparing spending differences across both regions and hospitals found that most of the spending was due to differences in use of the hospital as a site of care

(versus, say, hospice, nursing home, or the doctor's office) and to discretionary specialist visits and tests. Higher spending on these services does not appear to offer overall benefits. Other Dartmouth research suggests that hospitals spending more on effective care do in fact get better outcomes.

With the US figuring out how to provide health care coverage to millions of people who are uninsured, keeping care affordable matters, the authors wrote. Participants in the debate assume that growth in spending is inevitable and that it will be necessary to ration beneficial care:

> Neither of these conclusions is inevitable. Both rest on the assumption that all of the additional spending in high spending regions [or] areas is buying services that are necessary and beneficial. However, studies comparing similar patients have found that those in higher-spending regions are more likely to be admitted to the hospital, spend more time in the hospital, receive more discretionary tests, see more medical specialists, and have many more different physicians involved in their care. The extra care does not produce better outcomes overall or result in better quality of care, whether one looks at measures of technical quality (such as providing appropriate medication to heart attack patients), or survival following such serious conditions as a heart attack or hip fracture. Higher spending also does not result in improved patient perceptions of the accessibility or quality of medical care.[14]

The authors argued for limiting future spending increases by slowing the growth of capacity, getting better evidence on what works and using the payment system to reward value instead of volume.

As mentioned earlier, unnecessary care can come with serious risk to the person receiving it. Citing a *British Medical Journal* article, public health doctor Trevor Hancock wrote, "at least 250,000 Americans died in 2013 as a result of medical error, making it the third-largest cause of death after heart disease and cancer." In Canada, the Canadian Institute for Health Information has listed thirty-one types of harm that can occur in hospital, and in 2014–15 patients suffered potentially preventable harm in about one out of eighteen hospitalizations.[15] Some 70,000 Canadian hospital admissions each year are due to adverse events caused by the health care people have received, and for 1.6 percent of patients their death is associated with such an adverse event.[16] Besides the risk of harm to individuals, in Canada as in the United States, unnecessary care draws resources that could be better spent elsewhere.

The rapid growth in spending on health care services has been a big problem for many countries for many years. The editors of *Why Are Some People Healthy and Others Not?* (published in 1994) described the nature of health care funding debates as universally narrow. UBC health economist Robert Evans, Yale political scientist Theodore Marmor and UBC economist Morris Barer wrote about the battles for more money for health in the 1990s. "These contests centre on the familiar world of doctors and nurses, hospitals, and clinics. And they feature regularly the medical world's claim that more must be spent if the people (of Canada, the United States, France, Great Britain, Sweden, etc.) are to rightly enjoy the fruits of modern medical science."[17] The claims of "underfunding" have no relationship to the actual amount of money that is spent on health care, the authors wrote.

Over the decades, at least in Canada, health care spending has steadily risen. But that expansion hasn't necessarily made people healthier. As Andrew Thompson from the University of Oregon and Norman Temple from Athabasca University wrote in the introduction to *Exce$$ive Medical $pending: Facing the Challenge*, "The extravagance on healthcare spending might be justified if we could see clear evidence that it was directly responsible for major gains in the health of populations, but there is scant evidence of this."

Instead, they argued, better living conditions and healthier lifestyles have made a bigger difference. There had been medical successes, they allowed, including improved drug therapy for hypertension, cures for some cancers common in children, and advances in the treatment of traumatic injury. "But, on balance, medicine has promised far more than it has delivered, and it seems impotent in so many areas." They gave the example of obesity, which they called a pandemic sweeping the Western world. "Medicine has spent decades fighting the 'battle of the bulge,' but with virtually no success."[18]

They argued not for defunding health care, and not as others have for introducing a second tier where patients pay directly for some medical services, but for reducing waste so that more money would be available for other needs. "Our goal is to replace the current 'Rolls Royce medicine' with the development of a 'vw medicine,'" they wrote:

> Clearly, there is a yawning gap between expenditures deemed reasonable for normal living or affordable by average people and those deemed acceptable for medical procedures. It is as if the medical world is divorced from society and is living on another, far more opulent planet. The public, in effect, spends lavishly on medical care at the expense of its overall welfare.

That is, to extend their car metaphor, we are so strapped paying for Rolls-Royce medicine that we can't afford a healthy diet or a pair of jogging shoes in which to exercise. Luckily there's plenty of room in the back seat of the Rolls for sleeping. There were other options, they wrote, that could benefit many more people if the money were available. "Directing our resources to preventive-care programs would do far more for our health."

It's a phenomenon that's readily observable in British Columbia. In a March 2017 report the province's auditor general, Carol Bellringer, called attention to the ever-rising health care budget. Per person, the BC government spent $4,050 in 2016, which was slightly below the Canadian average. In a conference call with reporters, Bellringer said that the lower spending could be the result of a healthier population, but that it could also be the result of fewer services being offered. Despite spending less per person than other provinces, health was still by far the largest draw on BC's budget. The spending on health was already three times more than on education, the next largest ministry. And the increase the ministry was forecast to receive over a five-year period was equivalent to the entire budget of social development and social innovation, the third-largest ministry (see Figure 3.1). It was also equal to the money to be spent on the eleven smallest ministries.[19]

Fig 3.1   British Columbia Government Spending by Program Area

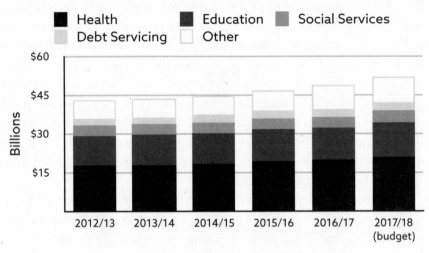

Source   BC Budget and Fiscal Plan 2017 September Update

Even within the health ministry's budget, some areas soaked up more spending than others. Since 2012, the amount spent on in-home nursing care had risen 14 percent. An extra 5 percent went to group homes for people with disabilities and residential care for seniors. Acute care—which includes emergency, post-surgical and critical-care services—was up 11 percent. The increase for services to help with mental health and substance use saw a smaller increase, just 3 percent. Meanwhile, tellingly, public health programs aimed at prevention, screening and controlling communicable diseases actually saw a decrease. For those programs, the budget was cut back by a percentage point.

"The health sector has the greatest spending pressure in all of government," Bellringer said. "While one-and-a-half percent here and three percent there may not seem like a notable difference, a one percent change to a major health program could be representing millions of dollars." I asked Bellringer how much sense it made to cut spending on prevention programs when they might offer a way to contain rising costs. She responded, "In terms of how much should be budgeted for an area, we leave that to the politicians. It's a policy call and it's actually something we're not permitted to comment on." But without telling them what to do, would more commitment to prevention not be a logical way to contain costs? "As a logical answer to that, of course, yes it would," she said. Bellringer pointed out that her office had previously warned the government what ever-rising health care costs could mean. "Rising health care costs may threaten the provincial government's ability to provide services and meet financial commitments, both now and in the future." Put another way, if health spending was allowed to continue rising rapidly it would reduce the government's ability to provide other services people need. It's a dilemma faced by governments across Canada and around the world.

In Canada, the authors of a report published in the CMAJ in early 2018 found that between 1981 and 2011 per capita spending on social programs had been flat while spending on health care had doubled. By 2011, provinces were spending about four times per person as much on health as they were on social programs. The priority was given to health spending despite the lack of evidence that it actually improved health. Meanwhile, the authors found, there is evidence that increased social spending improves health. "Population-level health outcomes could benefit from a reallocation of government dollars from health to social spending, even if total government spending were left unchanged."[20]

Decision makers need to balance the need to contain health care costs against the steady pressure to spend more. Sometimes that pressure comes from people who see their claim to those dollars as outweighing any other priority. As Thompson and Temple put it, funds are gobbled up for health care in part because of how people within the world of modern medicine see their profession. "A key problem with modern medicine is that it has set itself off from all other concerns," the two doctors wrote. "It has convinced itself that what it offers is so important that other concerns will just have to take care of themselves. It is not its problem if many people lack basic food, shelter, sanitation, and education, and that our basic provider, the environment in which we live, is dying." Instead, medical people tend to envision a future where ever more money is poured into technological improvements, they said. "It maintains its narrow focus on such pursuits as the need to develop more gene-targeted and mood-targeted drugs, and placing self-replicating neurons where they are needed, and then, somehow, everything will be much better, even though this pursuit drains the public coffers."[21]

Writing in *The New Yorker* magazine, the surgeon Atul Gawande gave a slightly different perspective on the successes of medicine, but also discussed the need to examine the expectations for health care. He wrote:

> We have a certain heroic expectation of how medicine works. Following the Second World War, penicillin and then a raft of other antibiotics cured the scourge of bacterial diseases that it had been thought only God could touch. New vaccines routed polio, diphtheria, rubella, and measles. Surgeons opened the heart, transplanted organs, and removed once inoperable tumors. Heart attacks could be stopped; cancers could be cured. A single generation experienced a transformation in the treatment of human illness as no generation had before. It was like discovering that water could put out fire. We built our health-care system, accordingly, to deploy firefighters. Doctors became saviors.

Gawande said that heroic role was part of why he wanted to become a surgeon in the first place; that ability to make an immediate difference for people is seductive. In the article, though, he contrasts that heroic self-image with the need for ongoing, long-term primary care that many conditions require. He gave the example of migraine headaches, and how it often takes many return visits to a doctor's clinic and gradual experimentation to discover how to help a particular patient. "If an illness is a fire, many of them require months or years to extinguish, or can be reduced only to a low-level smolder," Gawande wrote. "Much of what ails us requires a more patient kind of skill."[22]

There is, however, a huge market for faster results and there are companies keen to feed that demand. Often the high-tech fixes are pitched by people, especially in the pharmaceutical industry, who stand to profit from ever-increasing spending, according to Thompson and Temple. They highlighted the waste in some of the screening for cancer, genetic research and the wide use of statins. And they called for more rigorous assessment of new interventions. "What happens now is that procedures may become established on the basis of hope and low-grade evidence for their efficacy, and then gain organizational support for campaigns to make them standard, recommended offerings," they wrote. "It can even be considered unethical to subject them to rigorous criteria since that would deny some patients the chance to benefit from them. But the only sure thing about their effect is that the medical conglomerate makes a profit from using them." Those commercial interests find willing accomplices among politicians and other decision makers. "Medical research and treatment are routinely portrayed as crucial, life-saving activities, which elected officials dare not appear to be less than enthusiastic about," wrote Thompson and Temple.[23]

It is worth noting that the politicians must know that there is wide public support in Canada for health care spending and that it's clear who the people trust to manage that system. A June 2017 Insights West poll was typical in that it found that about 90 percent of Canadians had a positive opinion of nurses and doctors. The figure for politicians was 24 percent, held in lower esteem than lawyers, real estate agents, pollsters, car salespeople and even journalists.[24]

Drug spending is a particularly likely place to seek savings. Switching to lower-cost alternatives for some of the top prescribed drugs in Canada could reduce the amount spent by 55 percent, Temple wrote in a chapter of *Exce$$ive Medical $pending* written with Audrey Balay-Karperien and Joel Lexchin from York University's School of Health Policy and Management. Between 1996 and 2003 the country's spending on drugs had doubled, most of it to pay for high-cost, patented, highly marketed "me-too" drugs that offered no new benefit over existing products. "The Canadian public spends, directly or indirectly, almost a billion dollars a year in excess and unnecessary cash transfers to the pharmaceutical industry. And this figure will certainly be an order of magnitude larger in the USA," they wrote.[25] All of that money could be put to better use.

During a presentation to a House of Commons committee in Ottawa in late 2016, Tom Perry from the University of British Columbia's faculty of medicine, who is also a former MLA and cabinet minister, made the connection between high drug costs and the lack of money to address other contributors to good health:

> We should improve the health of Canadians, should not increase the harms, and should reduce drug costs and be proud of doing it, so that we can be sustainable and can fund the other determinants of health, such as clean water, proper nutrition, education, housing, and physical fitness, which are all suffering now in my province. We're spending so much money on health care, including drugs, that we no longer have music programs in our schools, for example. Also, as you know, we have many reserves all over the country without clean water.[26]

When we spoke in the summer of 2017, Perry was teaching clinical pharmacology and was involved in the Therapeutics Initiative, a research body that independently assesses drugs. In a phone interview, he gave the example of a muscle relaxant, cyclobenzaprine, that the Therapeutics Initiative was preparing a letter about. There's little evidence it helps and "it's probably mostly just harmful," he said. The drug is not licensed in Europe and is unavailable there, but in BC we spend $4 million a year on it, $1.5 million of that out of the public purse. The spending across Canada on the drug would be several times more.[27] "That's a trivial example," said Perry. Other similarly dubious drugs account for significant spending.

New drugs, particularly for "orphan diseases" that affect relatively few people, can cost hundreds of thousands of dollars a year.[28] While the evidence on whether or not they work can be mixed, there's often a push from those who feel they benefit to have them covered. Lilia Zaharieva, for example, a thirty-year-old in Victoria, received sympathetic media coverage as she sought to have the public PharmaCare plan pay for Orkambi, a drug for cystic fibrosis that Vertex Pharmaceuticals makes and sells for about $250,000 a year. "It's very painful to think about what it would be like to lose Orkambi," she was quoted saying. She had received funding for the drug through the insurance plan available to students at her university, but that was ending. "The feeling of watching these magical pink pills dwindle away every time I take them is both terrifying and yet a call to action."[29] The local paper characterized it as a "life-or-death fight" that could result in lung failure or the need for a transplant if unsuccessful. It was left to BC Health Minister Adrian Dix to explain that despite the "very serious situation," both Canada's Common Drug Review and the Drug Benefit Council had advised against funding the drug since they lacked evidence of its therapeutic benefits. The politician defending the decision, even though it is the responsible direction, risks appearing cold-hearted. And politicians face similar pressure across a wide range of diseases, often from patients' groups with strong ties to the drug industry.

As University of Victoria biomedical ethics professor Eike-Henner Kluge put it, "Clear thinking tells us that funding untried or unverified health care—health care that has not been shown to be more effective than other types of treatment (or no treatment at all)—is to fund on the basis of hope. Which is fine, when resources are unlimited." If resources are limited, then giving them to one person and not another needs to be justified, he wrote. "One should ask oneself … whether the particular individual for whom one is pleading is any more special than those others with whom one is not acquainted and of whose plight one is not aware."[30] With limited public funds available, there is a choice to be made between paying for an expensive, unproven drug, providing a family with housing, or raising ten families above the poverty line.

The public discussions about drugs like Orkambi don't tend to take into account what else the money might be spent on. "There is a profound bias toward prescribing drugs and other medical interventions," as Temple put it writing with Joy Fraser from the Centre for Nursing and Health Studies at Athabasca University. "In place of health promotion we have drug promotion!" Like Perry, they contrasted the demand for more drug spending with the fundamental problem that medical practitioners and governments tend to fail to recognize and embrace strategies for health promotion and illness prevention.[31]

A better approach would begin with recognizing the underlying causes of the majority of illnesses and proactively addressing them. As Temple observed, the key determinant of most of the major diseases afflicting Western societies is lifestyle. Cancer and heart disease have much more to do with smoking and diet, which are both closely tied to income, than they do with the care that's available. As Temple put it, "There is now very little debate that most of the diseases that afflict our society are preventable. It is impossible to exaggerate the importance of these medical findings, for they hold the key to effective action for disease prevention at the level of both the individual and the population." Prevention would in the long run be much cheaper than the current approach, he argued. "By its very nature, prevention is 'low-tech' and should therefore come with a modest price tag. Potentially, far more can be accomplished with far less resources than is typically the case with new 'high-tech' treatments." It's also better for the patient to avoid being sick in the first place. "Even when an effective treatment for a particular disease is available, it is obviously far better if we can prevent that disease, or at least postpone it until later in life."

There are many examples of prevention's past triumphs. Temple pointed to the success over the past 150 years fighting infectious diseases. "What is often forgotten is that primary prevention was the driving force behind this great success story," he wrote. "In particular, the widespread adoption of hygiene, after the importance of this was discovered, played a major role. Actual medical treatment, such as the development and use of antibiotics, played a fairly minor role." He referred to a 1998 study published in the *New England Journal of Medicine* that followed university alumni for more than three decades. The researchers found that those with a healthier lifestyle—defined as having a normal body weight, exercising and not smoking—lived on average an extra five years free of developing a disabling illness.

Temple was not, however, calling for a renewed commitment to pestering the population to make better choices. As noted earlier, deeper forces underlie the choices that individuals make. Here's how Temple put it:

> Clearly, a preventive approach to medicine holds tremendous potential. But equally clearly, there are enormous challenges to overcome, especially with respect to a general reluctance of large sections of the population to listen and follow the prevention advice. The rate of progress resembles a severely constipated

person who has taken a teaspoon of bran: things are moving, but very slowly.

Part of that slowness is due to the lack of control many individuals have over aspects of their physical environment, Temple acknowledged, giving the examples of pollution and food contamination. He could well have given smoking as another example, considering that the nicotine in tobacco is addictive. Temple argued that governments are in a position to prompt healthy behaviour in ways that go far beyond telling people to eat their vegetables. "Governments have the power to pass legislation and to manipulate prices using taxation and subsidies. These government powers have tremendous potential for influencing health behavior."[32]

Governments could also do more to set the conditions that would give more people the capacity to make better choices. In his 2012 book on the Canadian health care system, *Chronic Condition*, Jeffrey Simpson pointed out the need to combine health promotion with broader social supports. "If governments and their citizens were truly serious about health promotion, they would confront the social determinants of health, which would include employment and working conditions, housing, standards of living, early child development," he wrote. Efforts to promote healthier living and prevent illness have achieved little success because governments avoid acting on the link between the social determinants of health and health outcomes. "It is easier, and less costly, to develop health-promotion programs and to pursue a wellness agenda than to tackle entrenched income inequalities."[33]

Instead, health care soaks up every available dollar: "People can debate how those dollars should be spent within the health-care system, but they assume that health care trumps every public priority. Canadians, too, seem to think governments should spend more on health care, which means pushing more dollars into the system." But that might not be the wisest way to spend tax dollars, he said. "A dollar spent on poverty instead of the existing health-care system, or even some public-health programs, would be the best long-term investment not only in health but also in lessening cost increases," he wrote. It's a prescription that runs up against the perception that most people want health care now and are reluctant to see public money spent to relieve poverty. As Simpson put it, "The political reality of where dollars for health care have gone and will continue to go trumps the logic of where they should go."

No question we spend a heap of money on health care. In 2017–18, according to the federal budget, health transfers to the provinces and territories were to be $37.1 billion.[34] For British Columbia, spending on health was planned at $20.6 billion that year, a little more than four out of every ten dollars that passed through the government's coffers. And the amount was budgeted to grow by another $500 million in each of the following years. That adds up. If it was felt the money was being well spent, few would worry about it. But as André Picard put it in his 2017 book *Matters of Life and Death*, after adding in what provinces and territories spend, "Canadian health care is a $228-billion-a-year enterprise with no clear goals and a dearth of leadership. We talk endlessly about the sustainability of medicare but have no idea what we want to sustain."[35]

To many people, the prospect of better sustaining the health care system by spending more money to help people earlier seems counterintuitive. In his book *A Healthy Society*, Saskatchewan doctor and politician Ryan Meili made the case for more preventative care and broader social supports. "When we don't cover pharmaceutical costs or dental services, we increase costs not only for individuals, but for the system," he wrote. "As people are unable to pay up front, or if primary health services aren't available and accessible, they get sicker and present later in the course of their illness."[36] It would be much cheaper to prevent a disease like diabetes, or at least to identify and treat it earlier, than to pay for the long hospital stays and dialysis treatment that become necessary when the disease was caught too late to prevent kidney disease, Meili wrote. "Only by working on keeping people healthy can we hope to have a sustainable means of treating them when they are sick." Those practical arguments were on top of the moral ones, he wrote, including the indefensible idea that we will help people when they are sick and dying, but won't provide the resources to keep them healthy.[37]

The Public Health Agency of Canada put a price tag on health inequity in an April 2016 report. It used Statistics Canada data for 2007–08 and looked at services that make up about a quarter of health care provided in the country. As a person's income rises, both for men and women, the amount it costs to provide health care to them declines. "For the services included in this report, socio-economic health inequalities cost Canada's health care system at least $6.2 billion annually," the authors found. "This represents over 14% of total spending on acute care in-patient hospital-izations, prescription medications and physician consultations." In that inequity, however, they saw an opportunity. "There is potential to reduce these costs if all Canadians could match the health care usage patterns of the highest income group," they wrote. The biggest gains were to be found by improving the health of the people at the bottom of the income scale, the report said.[38]

A 2011 Canadian Centre for Policy Alternatives report found BC's health care budget could be trimmed by about 6.7 percent by providing more support to the province's poorest families.[39]

Samantha Nutt, a family physician and public health specialist who founded the group War Child Canada and served as its executive director, echoed that call to invest in what she called "hard to reach" populations, particularly for mental health. There's a need to get away from hyper-specialization so that people see doctors who can help them navigate the system, she said. "I would reinvigorate primary care." Beyond the health system, there's much that can be done as well. "We need to continue to have a very strong public education system because we know there's a close relationship between education and health ... All you have to do is look to the United States to see examples of where that is breaking down and in Canada we need to remember that too."

Within the management of health care, governments have a role as gatekeepers, making sure the public pays for what works and avoids wasting money on what doesn't. In doing so, more budget room would be created for needed action outside of the health care system, action with the potential to help many more people be healthier.

CHAPTER 4

Causes of the Causes
Living Conditions, Wealth and Status

On the map open on my computer screen, the Toronto neighbourhood where I grew up was pale yellow. The colour indicated that as in much of the north central part of the city, in Leaside the likelihood of dying early was relatively low. Meanwhile, a band of dark red ran across the city south of Bloor Street and the Danforth, stretching from downtown deep into the city's east end. In those and other red areas the chances of a premature death were two or three times as likely as in the yellow neighbourhoods (see Figure 4.1). The website for the Toronto Health Profiles Partnership had similar maps showing the uneven distribution of everything from chlamydia and diabetes to asthma and teen pregnancies.[1]

Other North American cities show similar patterns and in the United States, where economic inequality is greater and access to health care is worse, the divide is even more striking. In New York city, a person living near the 125th Street subway station in Harlem or the Elder Avenue station in the Bronx is twice as likely as someone on the Upper East Side or in Greenwich Village to have heart disease. Pre-term births happened 50 percent more often near Bronx and Harlem subway stations where the people are relatively poorer than they did in some of the richer areas. And people in the Bronx were 3.5 times more likely to be obese, itself a predictor of a host of illnesses, than were people near the 96th Street stop on the city's tony Upper East Side.[2]

In Chicago, the infant mortality rate near the Garfield stop in Washington Park on the city's south side is eight times what it is near the Armitage stop in wealthier Lincoln Park. Similarly, using 2009 figures, babies born near the Garfield stop were twice as likely to have a low weight at birth, which is associated with worse health. Children in that area were six times as likely to have elevated levels of lead in their blood as were children near Armitage. Coronary heart disease was more common in the poorer areas of Chicago as well.

The Robert Wood Johnson Foundation has published similar maps that the Virginia Commonwealth University Center on Society and Health created for more than twenty cities in the United States, all of which show how long people live is closely related to the economics of the neighbourhood where they live.[3] Life expectancy isn't the only measure that's important to people, but it is used as a rough indicator of health. And while many people might be accustomed to ignoring the inequalities in health, the neighbourhoods are often not in fact worlds apart. The poor lived as close as the rich to hospitals in many cases, but that availability did little to help them overcome the social and financial hurdles they faced in the rest of their lives.

The Robert Wood Johnson Foundation's website attributed the health gap in American cities to differences between neighbourhoods, including the education level of residents; income; having the tax base to support good schools; unsafe or unhealthy housing; access to nutritous food; and opportunities to exercise. "Proximity to highways, factories, or other sources of toxic agents may expose residents to pollutants," it said. Poor public transit could prevent residents from reaching good jobs, child care and social services.

Another US study found that men in the poorest areas died ten years sooner than men in the wealthiest ones. For women the difference was seven years. "The results should be deeply disturbing to all persons in the country," the authors wrote in the *American Journal of Public Health*. "Life expectancy in the poorest 'state' falls below that of more than half the countries in the world, meaning that, in essence, there are several developing countries hidden within the borders of the United States."[4] African-Americans who were not also Hispanic were 4.5 times more likely to live in the poorest areas than in the wealthiest.[5]

Fig 4.1 Toronto, Premature Mortality per 100,000 Population Age 0–74, Both Sexes, 2006–2008

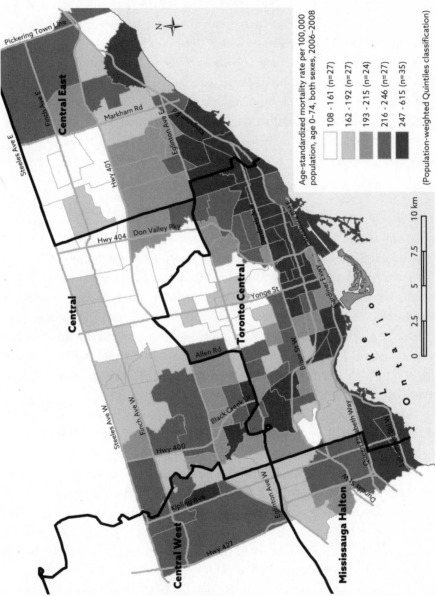

Source   Toronto Community Health Profiles Partnership, with data from
           Statistics Canada, 2006 Census of Canada and Ontario Mortality
           Data 2006–2008, Ontario Ministry of Health and Long-Term Care,
           IntelliHealth Ontario

As the economist Amartya Sen has put it, "Unnecessary suffering, debilitation, and death from preventable or controllable illness characterize every country and every society, to varying extents. As we would expect, the poor countries in Africa or Asia or Latin America provide crudely obvious illustrations of severe deprivation, but the phenomenon is present even in the richest countries. Indeed, the deprived groups in the 'First World' live, in many ways, in the 'Third.'"[6] Always with us, the poor and the rich are a few blocks or a short subway ride apart in many cities, just down the road in rural areas. But variations over time, or between jurisdictions, in the extent of poverty suggest there's nothing inevitable about it.

In Canada, where many are prone to smugness when it comes to comparisons with the United States, we have our own disparities. Among provinces, British Columbians live the longest (84 years for women; 81 for men) and people in Newfoundland and Labrador the shortest. Living on the west coast corresponds to three more years of life than people on the east coast get.[7] But people in the territory of Nunavut, where a significant proportion of the population is Indigenous, had the shortest life expectancy at birth in the country at 68.4 years for men and 72.9 years for women. According to Statistics Canada that's below the national average by 11.2 years for men and 10.9 years for women.

There are similar divides within the country when we consider conditions that affect people's quality of life. In terms of mental health, for example, Statistics Canada has reported that "In 2015, the likelihood of Canadians having contemplated suicide in the past 12 months varied by level of household income." For people over the age of fifteen who were living in households where the income was greater than $70,000, the number who had contemplated suicide in the past twelve months was 1.7 percent. In households where the income was under $20,000, the figure was more than three times higher at 5.8 percent.[8]

Even within relatively healthy British Columbia there are wide health inequities. Released in the fall of 2016, the My Health My Community survey of people in Vancouver found that the likelihood of someone saying their health was "good" or "excellent" was directly linked to which neighbourhood they call home. In West Vancouver, where most households have incomes over $100,000 a year, 73 percent said they were in "good" health or better. That rate was far higher than in poorer neighbourhoods, such as Strathcona, the area that includes Vancouver's Downtown Eastside and where the average household makes under $40,000 a year. There, only 34 percent of people, about half as many as in West Vancouver, said their health was "good" or "excellent."[9]

Across the province, people in richer areas outlive people in the poorest areas. People in the Lower Mainland and on southern Vancouver Island tend to be healthier than people in the northern and central parts of the province, according to a 2016 report from the Provincial Health Services Authority. "The results indicate more than a 10-year gap between the local health areas with the shortest and longest life expectancies," it said. Other worrying signs included that in the lowest income areas, kindergarten children were found to be the most likely in the province to be vulnerable in one or more of the five core areas of early childhood development. It also found:

> The rate of tobacco smoking is more than twice as high among adult British Columbians with less than high school education compared to those with at least a high school diploma, putting the first group at much higher risk for developing lung cancer and other chronic conditions. The rates of mood or anxiety disorder were more than twice as high among lowest-income British Columbians as compared to those in the highest income group.

The richest British Columbians did better than the poorest on many of the measures the report looked at. In its words:

> People in the highest income group reported significantly more favourable rates than those in the lowest income group for a number of indicators: positive perceived health (71.9% vs. 47.8%), positive perceived mental health (78.8% vs. 59.2%), adequate fruit and vegetable consumption (47.9% vs. 35.8%), leisure time

physical activity (69.3% vs. 48.2%), mood/anxiety disorder (7.9% vs. 17.4%) and current smoking (12.0% vs. 26.5%).

There were also gender differences, with adolescent girls reporting significantly higher rates of abuse and discrimination than boys, and "far fewer BC women than men reported that their health was 'excellent' or 'very good,'" the report said. "On the other hand, BC men reported much lower rates of adequate fruit and vegetable consumption than women, indicating an inequitable distribution of healthy eating habits."

The conditions people live in have a big influence on how healthy they are and the demands they're likely to make on the health care system, the report said. "We know that about 75% of our overall health is determined by social factors such as working or living conditions, income, and educational opportunities," wrote Lydia Drasic, then the executive director of the BC Centre for Disease Control Operations and Chronic Disease Prevention in the report's foreword. "These factors affect the rates of chronic disease and injury, contributing to health inequity or unfair differences in health and well-being for people of different groups." Those inequities came with a cost to the public and society at large, she wrote. "The direct health system costs associated with providing care to a sicker and more disadvantaged population are substantial. These costs are dwarfed by the indirect costs of health inequities, such as lost productivity, lost tax revenue, absenteeism, family leave, and disability or premature death." The report concluded that continued monitoring was needed to make it clear where inequities persist.[10]

Even once people are sick, wealth makes a difference. Ability to afford medicine, healthy food, rent, electricity and other necessities affects how well someone will be able to look after themself. Studies have shown that among people with diabetes, the poorest have a harder time managing with the disease than richer people do. Money even affects the likelihood that cancer treatment will succeed. For the wealthiest people living in Canada's cities, there's a 73 percent chance they will survive five years after they are diagnosed. For the poorest, the five-year survival rate is 61 percent. Put another way, if 100 rich people and 100 poor people are diagnosed with cancer, 12 more of the poor people than the rich will be dead within five years.[11]

One explanation for the differences in health outcomes involves material hardship. In testimony for the BC Utilities Commission about electricity rates in 2016, Emma Gauvin talked about how money affects people's health. She is the social work team lead for the STOP HIV/ AIDS program at Vancouver Coastal Health, which provides services to "Aboriginal people, LGBTQ2S (lesbian, gay, bisexual, transgender, queer/ questioning and two-spirited) communities, youth, immigrant and refugee communities, and people with mental health and/or addiction issues." She said, "We work with people who are HIV positive, and the majority of our clients struggle with addictions and mental health issues and have low incomes and live in unstable housing." That makes them vulnerable. "If someone is cut off by BC Hydro, then their lack of electricity becomes a priority. If our clients do not have electricity, this can derail treatment plans for other health issues." Clients who lose electricity in their homes risk having refrigerated and frozen food spoil, she said. "Many of our clients are prone to opportunistic infections, so not having access to proper nutrition can affect their health." Also, she said, two common drugs for HIV need to be refrigerated.

Or as Stacey Tyers, who manages counselling support services in Terrace and sits on the city's council, put it, "When it comes to low-income communities, every time there is a [hydro] rate increase, you are taking food out of someone's mouth." She described one client who lived in a trailer and faced a monthly BC Hydro bill of $300, a significant part of her budget. "She got to the point where she stopped buying her blood pressure medication so that she could keep up with her bills." Others avoid using power, Tyers said. "I know of many people that keep their heat well below where it should be in order to reduce costs," she said. "It is not healthy or safe for those people or their families. No one else would keep their heat that low."

Curtis Barton, a fifty-seven-year-old First Nations man living in Prince Rupert, testified, "After I pay my rent, I have $110 per month to spend on other expenses ... I have to choose between utilities and food. I have given up other expenses, including gas heating and internet in my home, and owning a car." Christopher Shay, a forty-three-year-old man who lives in Coquitlam and has been deaf since birth, said he forgoes other essentials so he can pay his electricity bills. "I do not have enough money left over each month to feed myself a healthy diet," he said. "I am six feet tall and I am often hungry."

Conrad Dennis, a forty-six-year-old First Nations man, was living on $610 a month in social assistance payments in Williams Lake. He lived with his mother, who was almost eighty and who he believed received a pension of about $1,000 a month, plus one other person. "I live with my mum as she has health problems, and I want to help her out," he said. Electricity is essential, especially since they heat with it, said Dennis. "It is really cold in Williams Lake in the winter. My mum is older, and she gets cold easily. She turns up the heat, and uses space heaters for a couple of hours each morning to heat up the house ... We can't really turn the heat down or off to save money, because my mom has a bad heart and brittle bones." He added, "I find it so stressful, and I get worried. I don't care so much about phone or lights, but we need heat—and my mom really needs a phone, lights, a fridge and heat."[12]

Unaffordable rents also suck up needed dollars. Of the 517,000 households that rent in BC, 70,000 of them spend 50 percent or more of their income on housing, Lorraine Copas, the executive director of the Social Planning and Research Council of BC told me. That level of spending makes a household vulnerable, she said. The number of people in that situation has been rising in recent years and includes 13,000 seniors, she said. "I would say we haven't necessarily gained ground at all."

David Hulchanski is a University of Toronto social work professor who specializes in housing. After a visit to Vancouver, where he had taught from 1983 to 1990 at the University of British Columbia, he said the city's street homelessness problem appeared to be getting worse. "It's quite appalling," he said. "The Downtown Eastside was frankly quite pleasant in the 1980s." While the neighbourhood was low income back then, there wasn't the same degree of chaos on the streets that exists now, he said. Hulchanski wrote a report in 1989 that found Vancouver's rental market was "collapsing," with the city's stock of good quality apartments in decline. "I think that report was a very specific warning about what was happening," he said. "After twenty-six years and 'the most successful housing strategy in North American history,' how many of the negative trends [and] problems have been taken care of?"

Lack of money can also affect whether someone takes medicine they've been prescribed. Research by Steve Morgan at the School of Population and Public Health at UBC and colleagues found that among residents of eleven wealthy countries, Canadians were the second most likely to skip filling a prescription. The survey found as many as one out of twelve Canadians failed to fill a prescription due to the cost. Using 2014 data from the Commonwealth Fund International Health Policy Survey of Older Adults, Morgan found that was worse than in Australia, France, Germany, the Netherlands, New Zealand, Norway, Sweden, Switzerland or the United Kingdom. The only country where the figure was worse was the United States, which lacks a publicly funded health care system and where one out of six said they skipped medicine due to cost.[13]

Statistics Canada found that, "Even in a system with universal health care, financial barriers may reduce access to medical care and can affect health outcomes." The study focused on people with chronic heart conditions, which can require long-term use of expensive medications, in the four western provinces. It found:

> Lack of drug coverage and general perceived cost barriers were reported by more than one in ten adults in western Canada with cardiovascular-related chronic conditions. These barriers were associated with lower use of guideline-recommended medications, an increased likelihood of non-adherence, and an increased likelihood of hospitalizations or emergency department visits.

Lack of drug coverage and the burden of co-payments and deductibles made it difficult for many to afford the drugs they'd been prescribed. "People with low socio-economic status are particularly vulnerable to experiencing poor health outcomes."[14]

In 2013, the Canadian Medical Association was estimating that social and economic factors determine 50 percent of health outcomes. The CMA divides the rest between health care (25 percent), genetics (15 percent) and your environment (10 percent). Gary Bloch, a doctor in family practice at St. Michael's Hospital in Toronto, has said, "Treating people at low income with a higher income will have at least as big an impact on their health as any other drugs that I could prescribe them ...

I do see poverty as a disease." Indeed, many of Canada's top causes of death have a significant social component, including many types of cancer, heart disease, stroke, accidents, diabetes and suicide. While they affect people at all income levels, they are more likely to affect people at the bottom. As part of his practice Bloch helps patients fill out applications and claim any provincial or federal support to which they might be entitled. "I absolutely see the improvement in my patients' health ... For patients that we do manage to get on income supports, their lives often really turn around."[15]

The words "poverty" or "social determinants of health" don't make it into the index of Timothy Caulfield's book *The Cure for Everything*, but the section on diet does make it clear that low-income families face added challenges when trying to eat well. "While the problem of obesity is not restricted to those in the lower socio-economic strata, numerous studies have found that it is more pronounced in lower-income groups. These groups typically have easy access to fast food while healthy options are harder to come by."[16]

No doubt being unable to afford healthy food makes a big difference to people's health. It comes with a range of risks, as Juha Mikkonen and Dennis Raphael wrote in *Social Determinants of Health: The Canadian Facts*:

> Dietary deficiencies—more common among food insecure households—are associated with increased likelihood of chronic disease and difficulties in managing these diseases. Heart disease, diabetes, high blood pressure, and food allergies are more common in food insecure households even when factors such as age, sex, income, and education are taken in account. Additionally, food insecurity produces stress and feelings of uncertainty that have health-threatening effects.[17]

The main determinant of how well a person eats is, of course, money. The Raise the Rates coalition has run the Welfare Food Challenge for several years. In 2016, for the fifth edition of the challenge, organizers calculated that after paying for rent and other essentials, a single BC welfare recipient would have $18 a week left for food. That works out to

$2.57 a day. For the 2015 report *Hungry for Justice: Advancing a Right to Food for Children in BC*, BC Civil Liberties Association researchers interviewed people in six BC communities. Lack of knowledge about healthy eating wasn't the problem, they found. Instead the report pointed to solutions such as increasing social assistance rates, raising the minimum wage and reducing the cost of other necessities like housing, transportation and child care. That is, people's food choices were closely tied to their economic circumstances. The rise of food banks over the last few decades, which fed 863,492 people in Canada in March 2016, also suggests many people can't afford food for themselves and their families.[18]

Ted Hawryluk, fifty-seven, a long-time recipient of disability benefits who lives in Victoria, told me that in 2015 the bulk of the $906 he received each month went to his rent of $706. It had gone up every year since 2007, a period over which his benefits had been frozen. Other expenses had gone up too. Between 2007 and 2014 the "all items" Consumer Price Index, which refers to eight major areas of spending that are considered necessities, such as food, shelter and clothing, rose by about 12 percent nationally and 8 percent in BC, according to Statistics Canada data. After rent, electricity and phone were deducted, Hawryluk was left with $56 a month. He has a degenerating bone disease that prevents him from doing the kind of physical labour he did when he was younger, but he netted about $12.50 a day selling the *Megaphone* street magazine. "I'm hungry most of the time," he said, adding he uses food banks and other charitable sources of food. He said he spends about $2 a day on ground beef. Asked whether he could make it by on just the government's assistance, he said, "I'd be dead of starvation. I'm a carnivore. I've got to have my meat."

To address hunger and other material deprivation, governments tend to focus on economic growth with the implicit promise that growth will lead to a better-off and healthier population. The evidence suggests, however, that increased economic strength does not on its own guarantee better health. Writing in *The Spirit Level: Why Equality is Better for Everyone*, Richard Wilkinson and Kate Pickett pointed out that countries do see gains in average life expectancy as national income grows, but only up to a point. People in poorer countries like Albania, Costa Rica and Uruguay have comparable life expectancies to people in Denmark,

Ireland and the USA, where incomes are four or five times higher. And during both world wars in the twentieth century, the people of Britain saw faster health gains than they did in times of peace. Wilkinson and Pickett attributed the unexpected health improvement to a decrease in inequality:

> A dramatic example of how reductions in inequality can lead to rapid improvements in health is the experience of Britain during the two world wars. Increases in life expectancy for civilians during the war decades were twice those seen throughout the rest of the twentieth century. In the decades that contain the world wars, life expectancy increased between 6 and 7 years for men and women, whereas in the decades before, between and after, life expectancy increased by between 1 and 4 years. Although the nation's nutritional status improved with rationing in the Second World War, this was not true for the First World War, and material living standards declined during both wars. However, both wartimes were characterized by full employment and considerably narrower income differences—the result of deliberate government policies to promote co-operation with the war effort.[19]

What matters is not how much economic activity there is, but how well the benefits are shared. A person's ability to afford food, medicine, a safe place to live and the other necessities of life have a direct impact on their health, but so does the sense of belonging that comes with a levelling of incomes.

Many of us respond to feelings of stress, emptiness or other emotions that come with inequality by making unhealthy choices. Only about 31.5 percent of Canadians over the age of twelve eat fruit and vegetables at least the recommended five times a day, suggesting that many who could afford to eat better do not.[20] Many who could buy apples find themselves drawn to the chip and soda aisle in the grocery store. George Orwell found "appalling" the diet of miners and their families in the north of England in the 1930s, but he was sympathetic to the choices they made. "The ordinary human being would sooner starve than live on brown bread and raw carrots," he wrote. "The peculiar evil is this, that the less money you have, the less inclined you feel to spend it on wholesome food. A millionaire may enjoy breakfasting off orange juice and Ryvita biscuits; an unemployed man doesn't."[21] The advertisers, of course, know how to take advantage of those feelings, and are at times identified as the villains in the story, far outspending governments or others hoping to encourage better choices.

Smoking, as well, can be understood as a choice people make in a social context. As University of Montreal sociology professor Marc Renaud put it, "Why would an individual deprive himself or herself of the pleasure of smoking if, on the other hand, his or her life is boring, work alienating, and prospects for the future either depressing or nonexistent? For some, smoking provides an admittedly dangerous but pleasant means to escape the stress and boredom of everyday life."[22] It's a perception backed up with statistics. In 2016 the Canadian Community Health Survey found smokers were about 50 percent more likely than non-smokers to report that most days were "quite a bit" or "extremely" stressful. They were also less likely to report being satisfied with their lives overall.[23]

The importance of "feelings" in this story speaks to a second explanation for why some people are healthier than others: the causes of illness are not just material, but social as well. So far I've focused on the fact that the health divide is greatest between the richest and the poorest. The gap between the extremes is stark and it's where the health inequities are most obvious. But it masks an important point: with each step down the income and social ladder, people are sicker. There are inequities not just between the very top and the very bottom, but between the people on the top and those on the rung immediately below them. People on the second rung are healthier than those below them as well, and so on down to the bottom. Put another way, even relatively well-off people who can afford nutritious food and a healthy home are likely to be sicker than people who are richer than them.

Michael Marmot, a professor of epidemiology and public health at University College in London, led some of the key studies demonstrating the links between people's social position and their health. They included the Whitehall Studies which found that among British civil servants, the lower they were in the hierarchy the more likely they were to get sick and the younger they were likely to die. In 2000 Queen Elizabeth knighted Marmot for his contributions.

Marmot was the chair of the World Health Organization's Commission on Social Determinants of Health when it was active between 2005 and 2008. Describing his work for the WHO in an interview posted on the international body's website, Marmot made an international comparison:

> Let's start at the beginning: if you are a fifteen-year-old boy in Lesotho, your chance of reaching the age of 60 is about 10%. If you are a fifteen-year-old boy in Sweden, your chance of reaching 60 is 91%. This difference is due to social conditions, which are determinants of health. They include education and the nature of jobs. They include living conditions such as housing and availability of adequate nutritious food. They also entail access to quality health care.[24]

Within countries there are also large health inequalities, Marmot said. Giving the example of the United States, he pointed out that life expectancy in downtown Washington, DC, is fifty-seven years, while in the Maryland suburbs a short train ride away it is seventy-seven years. "There is [a] 20-year life expectancy [gap] in the nation's capital, between the poor and predominantly African American people who live downtown, and the richer and predominantly non-African American people who live in the suburbs," Marmot said. "Now, a poor man in inner-city Washington, D.C., is rich in material terms when compared to a poor man in Lesotho. The social determinants of these two individual's lives are different, and we must acknowledge this and think of poverty in a different way." Health is not then just about the food and material goods a person can afford. Marmot said, "It is about opportunities in life and control over one's life, in addition to social conditions that shape the physical environment one lives in."

In Canada, a 2013 study illustrated the point well. Statistics Canada researchers looked at the health of 2.7 million Canadians over a sixteen-year period, dividing them into five groups, or quintiles, based on income.

Fig 4.2   **Premature Deaths, Canada, by Income Quintile**

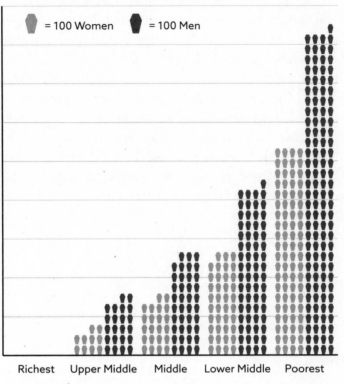

If everyone were as healthy as the top 20 percent, there would be 40,000 fewer deaths each year, they found. The gap in health was largest between the lowest quintile and the one just above it, but there were also gaps between each group. According to calculations researcher Michael Tjepkema provided by email, roughly 20,000 of the extra deaths would be of people in the lowest income group. But there would also be 10,355 deaths in the second-lowest group and 6,020 in the middle income group. Even the group right below the top earners would have 3,180 fewer deaths if they were as healthy as people in the top group (see Figure 4.2).[25]

Writing in the *Toronto Star*, York University health policy and management professor Dennis Raphael and Toba Bryant, an assistant professor of health sciences at the University of Ontario Institute of Technology, suggested that the number of deaths from health inequities that the Statistics Canada study had identified was comparable to having a plane crash killing 110 passengers in the country every single day. And yet, nobody seemed to care.[26] There is something obviously unfair about a society where despite valuing universal access to health care your likelihood of being sick or well depends largely on your income and your social position. In some cases the inequities are difficult to observe at the individual level, but in other cases they exist in plain view. Certainly that's the case with the interlinked crises in mental health, addictions and housing with which many people struggle. What should be viewed as health issues instead tend to become a problem of public disorder for local officials to manage.

CHAPTER 5

Worrying Symptoms
Mental Health Care
and Tent Cities

Zeb Baranyai was uncertain what was wrong with him. "I just feel this deep sense of fear or sorrow," he told me. He frequently breaks down in tears or feels inexplicably sad. Other times, his illness feels more like anxiety or is expressed as anger. Without warning, the feelings boil over. "There's no filter or progression that I can see," he said. "I hesitate to say 'out of control,' but I feel like I'm someone else in those moments."

We were meeting on a sunny spring day in a Victoria coffee shop and Baranyai's former partner, Sarah Grantham, was with us. Hand wrapped around the handle of a mug, she looked at him. "You are out of control in those moments," she said. She's seen Baranyai, a physically strong man in his thirties, break phones, computers and tables, she added. She's felt unsafe. "This is not run-of-the-mill depression. There's something else going on. It's not healthy behaviour and anyone who took the time to listen would realize it's not healthy behaviour." They'd recently begun living separately so that they could each better look after themselves.

When we met, Baranyai had already spent a year trying to get help dealing with his mental illness. "I feel shuffled around," he told me. "I don't have what I need. I'm just trying to access the help that's available to me." While waiting for care he'd lost a good job with a computer software company and was having a tough time making ends meet.

The waiting had made what would have been a difficult time worse, Grantham said. "It's just been really terrible. It's just been a total shit show."

For ten months Baranyai had been waiting to have an MRI scan of his brain and it takes over a year to see a neuropsychiatrist, Grantham said. He had been seen by Island Health's Urgent Short Term Assessment and Treatment program, which promises on its website "short-term individual psychotherapy for patients in crisis, at risk, or in severe distress." But Grantham said appointments tend to be for thirty minutes every six weeks. "It feels like they're going through the motions," she said. "There's nothing 'urgent' about it."

Baranyai said he wondered if what he was experiencing was related to past concussions. "A diagnosis of some sort would be helpful for me," he said. Instead he was without a clear idea of what was wrong or how to go about getting better. Though he had taken drugs he'd been prescribed for depression and anxiety, he said, "There's nothing that I'm working towards that I can tell." Baranyai, who has a university degree in sociology and social justice, said his inability to get help isn't unusual. "My experience is not unique to me. I know this is happening to other people."

Indeed, such stories are easy to come by. A Victoria optometrist participating in the Canadian Mental Health Association's Ride Don't Hide event highlighted in a widely shared email how hard it can be to get help. "As a well-documented person with mental illness I can tell you that resources like those provided by this organization are sadly lacking," wrote Neil Paterson. "These services are barely available to people of means, I can't imagine being mentally ill and poor in Victoria."

And it took five years for Christianna Shand, a Fort St. John teacher, to get help for her daughter who at five years old began expressing a desire to commit suicide. The treatment was good when she was eventually admitted to the BC Children's Hospital in Vancouver, said Shand, but it was a fight to get there. "It was years of work that I did." Her daughter, who was eventually diagnosed with bipolar disorder, was seen for a while by a counsellor with child and youth mental health services. "They saw her, but they were really strapped for resources," Shand said. Eventually her daughter was "kicked out" for not meeting the program's criteria, Shand said, forcing her to pay privately for care. "She really did have a problem," she said.

A 2016 report out of Manitoba noted, "Canadian studies suggest that 1 in 7 children experience mental disorders at any given time, however less than a third of these children receive the clinical treatment services they require."[1] The Canadian Mental Health Association says that in any given year, one out of five Canadians will experience a mental health problem or illness. It's an experience that half of the people in the country will either have or have had by the time they are forty years old. In many of those cases, people will spend years seeking help. Care can be particularly hard to find for people who are unwell but not yet in crisis.

Former Victoria dental surgeon David Heft wrote in a local newspaper about struggling with depression and anxiety for thirty-two years. "It is now apparent that the system is becoming designed to deal with extremes, and those of us who are not perceived to be 'sick enough' for care (at that moment in time) are being ignored," he wrote. "I have seen too many individuals sent home by Island Health because the psychiatric emergency room was too small and there were far too few psych inpatient beds to deal with the needs of a large city such as Victoria. The destructive consequences of having to go through an episode outside of a safe environment is irreparable, not only to the patient but also to those who have the misfortune of having to deal with the broken pieces." The health authority was pulling funding for the support group he was in, he said. "By removing services, a large segment of the population will be forced to be seen by walk-in clinics and family physicians where psychiatric care that is called for is not provided. In fact, many do not even have a physician, let alone a psychiatrist, which often leads to the police force having to deal with their mental-health issues."[2]

In February 2017, CBC reporter Curt Petrovich described on the radio show *The Current* how difficult it was to find treatment for the post-traumatic stress disorder he'd developed covering disasters like typhoon Haiyan in the Philippines in 2013 for the public broadcaster. Living in Vancouver, he was told it would take a year to see someone who could treat PTSD, he said. "That's what I was facing. I was basically told that I have a mental illness that needs to be treated but there really is nobody that can treat you." The only way he got help, which involved lots of talk therapy over a period of months, was by entering a study using the drug MDMA, better known as ecstasy, for treatment. "If I hadn't been [in the study], I don't know where I'd be today," Petrovich said. His wife, Yvette Brend, said, "It is impossible to find help for PTSD. There is nothing out

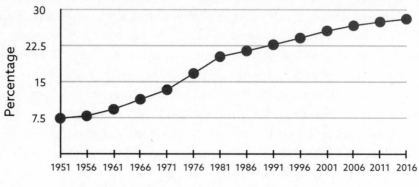

Fig 5.1 **Percentage of One-Person Households, Canada, 1951 to 2016**

Source   Statistics Canada, Census of Population, 1951 to 2016

there for families specific to PTSD. And we live in a have province where you'd think there'd be a lot, but it's really difficult to find support."[3]

Jonny Morris, the senior director for policy at the BC division of the Canadian Mental Health Association, told me he was not surprised by stories of people suffering while they waited a long time to get help. "We do have very fragmented care. There are gaps in care. It is sometimes quite tricky to find everything you need." The public health care system fails to cover psychotherapy, he said, and the available mental health services are more oriented towards crisis care than community-based interventions that could better support people earlier. Problems are allowed to fester into crises before help is given.

The connection between a person's social circumstances and their health is perhaps easiest to see when we consider isolation, a condition that cuts across the population. Figures from the 2016 Canadian census showed that the 28.2 percent of households that consisted of a single person was the highest it had ever been and had for the first time become the most common type of household in the country (see Figure 5.1). That rate was similar to the rate in the United States and the United Kingdom, but not as high as France, Japan, Sweden or Germany, where 41.4 percent of households in 2015 included just one person.[4] In a 2016 piece published a few days before Christmas, Massachusetts physician Dhruv

Khullar described the heartbreak of treating patients who were alone over the holidays, as well as during the rest of the year. "Social isolation is ... increasingly recognized as having dire physical, mental and emotional consequences," he wrote. "Individuals with less social connection have disrupted sleep patterns, altered immune systems, more inflammation and higher levels of stress hormones." Isolation increases the risk of heart disease by 29 percent and stroke by 32 percent according to one recent study, Khullar wrote. "Another analysis that pooled data from 70 studies and 3.4 million people found that socially isolated individuals had a 30 percent higher risk of dying in the next seven years, and that this effect was largest in middle age." Many studies have found that social connections and good marriages have protective effects.

The effects of isolation are long term and start young, said Khullar. "Socially isolated children have significantly poorer health 20 years later, even after controlling for other factors," he wrote. "All told, loneliness is as important a risk factor for early death as obesity and smoking." Despite the risk, stigma can make it extremely difficult for people to seek help, said Khullar. "Admitting we're lonely can feel as if we're admitting we've failed in life's most fundamental domains: belonging, love, attachment."[5]

In a discussion paper for the Columbia Institute in Vancouver, researchers Gloria Levi and Laura Kadawaki wrote about the substantial evidence linking health and social isolation:

> Socially isolated seniors are more at risk for falls, not eating well, and sedentary behaviour. Isolation is even a predictor of mortality from coronary disease and stroke, and isolated seniors have a four to five times greater risk of hospitalization. Social isolation also affects the psychological and cognitive health of seniors, such as depression and suicide. Ironically, the cause of death of socially isolated seniors is often stated as "failure to thrive."

They saw a role for local governments to provide diverse programs through community centres to help counteract the effects of isolation. Those programs could include ones aimed at improving physical well-being, such as fitness, nutrition and health promotion, as well as ones supporting creativity and intellectual development. Opportunities to volunteer would help people feel needed and like they belong, they wrote. "With the mounting cost of our present health care system, there will be an increasing focus, expansion, and funding of community-based health care," they wrote. "Municipalities need to see the role seniors' programs play within this continuum. These programs play a central role in wellness promotion."[6]

The need is there in part due to the stingy way we provide mental health care in Canada, which is itself symptomatic of a much wider public policy failure. On any number of fronts—think social housing, First Nations' education, childcare, early learning and welfare systems—our representatives make pinching pennies the priority. But by doing so we at times trade short-term savings for long-term consequences that can lead to the public—as well as individuals—paying a much higher price later.

That day with Baranyai in the Victoria coffee shop, Grantham hit on a prime example. The way she sees it, she said, untreated mental illness is a root cause of homelessness. A stronger mental health system could greatly reduce the number of people who end up in that kind of deep crisis, she said. At the time, the British Columbia capital, a generally peaceful place of lush gardens and progressive thinking, was host to a tent city of more than a hundred people who were homeless. The encampment on the downtown courthouse lawn was testing the patience of neighbours, who complained about theft, mess and disorder. Politicians were under increasing pressure to disperse the camp. Grantham, though, looked to the camp's roots. Many of the people living there were suffering, she observed. "If there was better mental health services in BC, then people in tent city wouldn't be there."

As it happens, a few months earlier, I'd taken the opportunity to visit the tent city myself and meet some of the people living there. One of them was Norm Ruble, a thirty-two-year-old who grew up in Vancouver. He told me a story about the tent city that was somewhat more complicated. It involved mental health, drugs and limited options, sure, but ultimately it came down to money.

Ruble had been living in what its residents called Super InTent City for several months and said it beat living away from the city centre in isolated parks, where the police enforce a city bylaw that requires tents to be taken down at 7:00 each morning. "I'm going to choose the group [living] outside of the courthouse every time," he said. He'd been living outside for about a year and a half. Before that, he was housed in a building run by the Victoria Cool Aid Society for people who are hard to house, but that ended badly. He regularly butted heads with the group's employees, he said, over what seemed to him like arbitrary rules. "Random stuff, [like] saying friends of mine can't bring their backpacks upstairs, to my house."

Ruble said one day a housing employee believed him to be under mental duress and called the police. "When they entered my house they pretty much grabbed me right away and said 'stop resisting' and threw me around, punched me in the head, dropped knees on my chest. I had fractured ribs from that." The officers claimed they thought Ruble was reaching for a knife, Ruble said. When it went to court, the judge sided with the officers. Ruble was found guilty of "wilfully resisting or obstructing a peace officer," and his sentence included a ban from being within a block of any Cool Aid properties, resulting in him becoming homeless. A spokesperson for Cool Aid took questions but said for privacy reasons nobody from the agency would comment.

For Ruble, becoming homeless at first seemed like a good option. "I chose to become homeless because well, I was just sick and tired of life the way it was for me, and honestly it's very, very freeing when you become homeless for the first time. Not needing to pay rent on anything, not needing to worry about having to work for this, work for that."

Ruble said before living in a tent he'd been stressed about money all the time. "I'd also just been charged with uttering threats. That caused me to lose my security job ... For the line of work I was doing, yeah, [you] couldn't really have a record for it."

Camping on public property is legal in Victoria due to a 2008 ruling that found it unconstitutional to prevent people who are homeless from sleeping on public grounds or erecting shelter to protect themselves when there are not enough shelter beds available for the number who are homeless. The city bylaw that requires tents to be taken down during the daytime doesn't apply at the courthouse since the location is private property belonging to the provincial government.

To their residents, tent cities can be a better option than a shelter or a downtown doorway. "It's kind of a surprising thing for a man to call a tent on a lot his home, but it's more than just a tent somewhere," camper Nicholas Jewell said. "All these people have set up their shelters and the reason is a lot of the solutions offered … just don't fit these individuals. Some people are happy outside. Some people don't like the rules and regulations put down by shelters. Some people don't like the health risks shelters do present." The camp is a community, said Jewell. "Together we can keep an eye on each other, we can cover each other's weaknesses and let our strengths grow so we become something more than just the individuals," he said. "We've got each other's backs here."

To critics, tent cities are a symptom of failed public policy. As Stephen Portman, the advocacy lead at the Together Against Poverty Society in Victoria, put it one day standing in the dust amid the tents, "Instead of displacing a tent city, we're asking the government to end the conditions that require a tent city." Noting BC has also seen tent cities arise in Abbotsford, Maple Ridge and Surrey in recent years, Portman said, "They are a product of a disappearing social safety net and thirty years of disinvestment in social housing, shameful welfare rates and disability and pension rates, and a government that is truly failing its people."

When I saw Ruble again a couple months later, on a day when provincial government lawyers were pressing in British Columbia Supreme Court to remove the tents from the lawn outside, he was positive. "Having a place to sleep every night is great," he told me. "Just having a place for my stuff and to lay my head at night has been doing wonders for me. I bet I look a lot more healthy, too. I feel a lot more healthy."

Ultimately though, living outside was getting tiresome and he wanted to find a place indoors. "After so many years being homeless, on the street and what not, no, I want a house. I want a house again. This is great for now, but we all know this tent city's not going to last, then from my point of view it's going to be right back to 7 a.m. wake-up calls."

Asked how drug use in the tent city compared to elsewhere on the streets, Ruble said, "Right about the same level. Everyone's addicted. There's no more drug use, less drug use. The addicted will go for what they want." He figured that addiction was relatively minor in the list of causes behind the tent city. "There are so many functioning users who you'd never suspect," he said. "I've had friends who were able to go to work completely rocked on morphines or whatever their drug of choice is, whatever that may be, they've been able to go to work, work, do their job, come home, get more, be a totally functioning drug addict. Sure, for some people, certain situations, that can be a cause for homelessness, but it's not that big of a factor."

His observation rang true. In middle-class neighbourhoods like mine, there are plenty of people who indulge in drugs or alcohol in the privacy of their own home, and still make it to work in the morning. In 2013, according to the most recent figures available on the government of Canada's website, some 458,000 Canadians, or about 2 percent of the population, reported they'd used at least one of cocaine, crack, speed, ecstasy, hallucinogens or heroin in the previous twelve months.[7] And 5.5 million Canadians over the age of twelve, almost 19 percent of us, that year reported high enough alcohol consumption to be considered heavy drinkers.[8]

So, I asked Ruble, really it's about money? He responded, "It's always money."

That there's something deeply wrong in North American society is obvious. We produce an endless stream of broken people, surplus to the job market, who struggle with mental illness, addictions and keeping a home. While it's possible for some in our rich society to ignore the problem, and many do, dealing with the resulting disorder often becomes the responsibility of municipal politicians. They hold few of the levers that would affect the flow of the stream, and few resources for mopping it up, yet find themselves left to do just that. So it was for good reason that tent cities and the underlying issues were top of mind at the annual Union of British Columbia Municipalities convention in 2016. The annual meeting gathered mayors and councillors from across the province in Victoria, as well as provincial politicians and staff members from both levels of government.

Nicole Read, the mayor of Maple Ridge, spoke on a panel one morning about the challenges her city faced when a tent city mushroomed on a residential street in 2015. Around forty years old, Read was a relatively young mayor. Her biography on Maple Ridge's website said, "My younger brother and I were raised by a single mother and we grew up well loved but quite poor."[9] When she spoke, Read said that Maple Ridge, with support, responded to its tent city without resorting to the legal system to disband the encampment and found housing for 143 people, all but 13 of whom remained housed. Some 189 people were referred to mental health services, 89 to detox and 71 to treatment for addictions. They'd had success, Read told the crowded auditorium, but the point she really wanted to make was about the drivers of homelessness. "We have a younger than average regional population of homeless people between the ages of 19 and 35 who are extremely street entrenched," she said. "They are heavily addicted, they are severely mentally ill, and it's very difficult to connect some of these people to housing."

Creating a National Housing Strategy, a process started after Justin Trudeau's Liberals were elected federally in 2015, is important but not enough on its own, she said. "We have to get upstream and invest in our kids. We absolutely have to prevent our kids from entering pathways that lead to homelessness." There are many vulnerabilities, she said. "We don't have enough community based resources ... We've got a lack of school councillors, children who have increased anxiety."

There are too few residential treatment beds for young people with addictions, and statistics from the Kids Help Phone say that one out of five youth seriously considered suicide in the last twelve months, Read said. "If we can't keep our kids from feeling vulnerable, then when drugs are introduced to them we will continue to see kids enter the pathways that lead them to the streets," she said. While some in the community still believe in promoting abstinence from all drugs, it's clear that approach will continue to result in more youth becoming homeless, she said. "We need to treat this as a health issue and not a moral issue."

Maple Ridge and other municipalities are paying to deal with problems they've inherited. A 2014 Columbia Institute report called *Who's Picking Up the Tab?* found that as federal and provincial governments shirk their responsibilities, local governments find themselves "picking up the slack on housing, mental health, addiction, social services" and more.[10] Responsibilities resulting from the deinstitutionalization of people suffering from mental illnesses and the decline in housing support add costs for local governments, the level least able to pay, the Columbia Institute's executive director, Charley Beresford, told me.

Speaking on the UBCM convention panel, Victoria Mayor Lisa Helps said, "Tent cities are expensive." Cities like hers have been saddled with that expense in part due to the federal government's shifting priorities: in 1989 the federal government spent $114 per Canadian on housing, she said, a figure that had dropped to $58 by 2014.

After the panel, I found Read and asked her to talk more about what her city had been dealing with. She explained that many of the young people on Maple Ridge's streets had challenges as adolescents that were never properly addressed. Many were addicted to opioids and struggling with mental health:

> I've had this conversation with our school district, which is one of our biggest partners in all of this conversation about youth. When you've got a large number of foster homes in your city, and these kids have to go to school and you don't have mental health resources and supports in the school, and you've got eight months to a year wait times around public access to psychiatric services or psychological services, it's a real problem.

Maple Ridge had been paying to bring a psychiatrist out from Vancouver once a week, but after an initial drop, the wait-list had begun to grow again. Read said her city needed a dedicated youth mental health clinic. "Ultimately it's a provincial health issue and we need to tackle it as a health issue," she said.

When I asked Read what she'd like to see done differently, she said she would start with making changes to the education system. For many kids who might not be getting support at home, supportive teachers are essential, she said. "The first line of defence is our school system. Teachers there, they love their kids and they're with them every day. They know when something's wrong. The challenge I think for a lot of our teachers right now is they don't have the ability to do anything and it's so frustrating for them." Also, fewer kids with disabilities and challenges are being identified, so many are not getting the treatment they need, she said.

"We had a number of Aboriginal people on our streets ... The residential school system has an impact and a disastrous legacy because you have kids who were taken out from families who've never been parented who don't learn how to parent. We see the lasting consequences from that in families and it's going to take time certainly to heal that."

Ultimately, said Read, success will depend on confronting the issues with open hearts and to work on them consistently. "I believe fundamentally that we need to approach people with compassion. I have this understanding that a lot of things go wrong in a person's world to lead them to the street. We have to meet them where they are and we have to be kind. We gain nothing by not being kind." The public is in many cases far from compassionate on the issue, however, Read acknowledged, which is a challenge for a politician. "It's very difficult to navigate the public sentiment around this issue and to not become demoralized, but we need people to be champions and continue to just see the end goal and work towards the end goal," she said.

Vancouver Councillor Kerry Jang is also a psychologist and teaches psychiatry at the University of British Columbia. We sat and talked on a couch in the bright lobby of the Empress Hotel, which adjoins the conference centre in Victoria. Vancouver's homeless population has been becoming younger, he observed. Factors include the lack of support for people leaving prison, aging out of government care or arriving from other provinces. A huge number of people who are homeless come from First Nations, he said. "Every story is individual," he said. "It's always a confluence. People's reasons for falling into homelessness are varied." The response needs to be varied as well, he said, pointing out the need to increase shelter allowances, extend foster care so people over nineteen years old remain supported, and address poverty. When 53 percent of the people in the province are living paycheque to paycheque, as a 2016 survey had found, many people are vulnerable, he said.

When it comes to protecting kids from drug addiction, an opportunity for them to see the consequences helps, said Jang. Many parents talk about sheltering their children from the reality of the crisis playing out in Vancouver's Downtown Eastside, but not Jang, who visited Chinatown and the Downtown Eastside with his kids from when they were very young. "They saw how you walk through there. You walk, you say 'hi' to folks if they say 'hi' to you, you treat them like they're human, and guess what, you're going to be fine." By 2016 Jang's kids were university aged.

"I took them down there at a very young age, and they never expressed an interest [in drugs] … If we want to inoculate our kids, just teach them. It's not about prohibition, but here are the pros and cons, here are the choices."

Jang said he had long been an activist, but got into politics because it was a way to bring in different areas of expertise to hopefully make a difference for people. "When you think of medicine, psychology, psychiatry, all the helping professions, it's all very much focused on individuals. It's almost focused on the individual at all costs, not realizing there are other issues out in the world. As a politician, putting that hat on, I've come to realize there's a whole other world out there I never knew existed." Individuals live in a social context and there's need for a systemic approach that would prevent them from needing more help later.

Rich Coleman was another politician who appeared to have glimpsed that other world. At the time he was the cabinet minister responsible for housing, as well as the natural gas minister and the deputy to then premier Christy Clark. Speaking on the UBCM panel on homelessness and tent cities, he said, "The biggest challenge is, how do we stop these in the future?" He observed, "There's an underlying challenge here, it's a social challenge and it's pretty dramatic."

Later I met Coleman in a hallway and had a chance to ask what he meant when he talked about the social crisis underlying the growth in tent cities. He said, "There are so many multiple barriers and there are so many underlying social issues. That's why we put outreach workers into shelters and on the streets." In some cases the issue might be literacy, in many others it's mental health, he said. "Other stuff gets more complicated when you have mental illness and drug addiction, that type of stuff together." There's a need to provide "wrap-around" services that provide for people's basic needs, including housing and food, said Coleman. "Once you get them the nutrition side you can work on getting their head straight enough that they can go deal with some of the others," he said. Not everyone responds well to harm reduction, but the government was trying to help people stabilize so they could receive help. "It's all a big social interaction."

When I later told NDP leader John Horgan about Coleman's comments, he said the provincial government had long been ignoring its own role in creating the crisis. It's true the province had done little to avoid more people hitting bottom. Child poverty had been allowed to spike and remained higher than the Canadian average. That poverty was itself a reflection of failures to set the conditions that would allow families to thrive as the government gave tax cuts priority over providing services. After 2001 the minimum wage dropped from among the highest in the country to the lowest. Welfare rates were frozen for a decade. Horgan, who would become premier following the 2017 election running on a platform to make life more affordable, strengthen government services and make the economy more inclusive, said, "It's that underlying social problem they don't seem to get. There is no mental health and addictions system in British Columbia ... Clearly [there's] a crisis in our mental health and addiction services here in British Columbia." First responders were dealing with the brunt of it, and there was a failure to fix the problem at the root, he said. "Once you get someone back up on their feet, you're not going to get them back into the community unless they have access to services. That's treatment beds, and that means rehabilitation and recovery houses, that's the challenge. The government's fallen well short of the demand there and I think they need to do more."

The failure to be proactive leads to later costs for governments. Tent cities and homelessness, for example, are themselves expensive. What governments save by failing to support Ruble and others, to avoid them becoming homeless, they end up spending in other ways. The province spent $3 million on the Victoria tent city, the local newspaper reported long after it ended. The expenses included almost $800,000 in legal fees and $1.7 million for garbage removal, water, hydro, fencing and security. As well, the city boosted its policing budget by $113,000 due to the camp and BC Housing's costs included paying for temporary shelter.[11]

When considering the true cost to society of tent cities, the expense needs to be multiplied across the many communities that host such encampments. A February 2017 report from Metro Vancouver found there were seventy homeless camps across the region. An estimated 4,000 people were in immediate need of housing and for six years the number of unsheltered homeless people had been rising by 26 percent per year. "Approximately five additional people will become homeless within the region each week, while more than 60,000 households in Metro Vancouver spend more than half their income on shelter, making them vulnerable to homelessness," the city's Regional Homelessness Task Force found. "Homelessness has increased steadily in Metro Vancouver over the past 15 years, driven by major gaps in social services for people with chronic health issues, mental illness or addictions, and exacerbated by the meteoric rise in rents, house prices and the cost of living."[12]

Across Canada in 2016, an estimated 35,000 people were homeless on any given night and 235,000 would be homeless at some point during the year.[13] In the United States, on one night in January 2016 a national survey estimated there were more than 560,000 people homeless, with the problem particularly entrenched in the western states.[14, 15]

In Vancouver, the city calculated it was spending $55,000 a year per homeless person. Housing them would cost $37,000. It called on senior levels of government to help with a plan to prevent people from becoming homeless, serve those who are homeless and find them ways into housing. Priorities included more transitional housing for foster youth, home care for people with mental illnesses and addictions, and creating new affordable and social housing units.[16]

The Metro Vancouver report included some interesting clues about the roots of the crisis. Forty percent of the homeless had previously been in the criminal justice system and a similar number had been in government foster care. Four out of five had a chronic health issue, about a third had a mental illness and half had an addiction. Critically, 70 percent of the people who were homeless reported they'd experienced trauma or abuse in the past. As I'll discuss in more detail in chapter 7, Indigenous people were over-represented. An earlier Canadian Mental Health Commission study followed nearly 600 homeless people over two years and found 67 percent had at least two mental illnesses or addictions.[17]

The guiding principles outlined in Vancouver's report included the observation that preventing homelessness was easier than reversing it and would be better for residents and taxpayers over the long term.

It's not just the streets where people with mental illnesses are over-represented. As André Picard notes in his book *Matters of Life and Death*, "Of those sentenced to a federal penitentiary (meaning sentences of two years or more), one in four has a diagnosed mental illness, and 80 percent have a serious substance-abuse problem. Federal penitentiaries and provincial jails (as well as our streets) have become de facto mental institutions." It's a failure three decades in the making, he wrote. "In the 1970s, Canada had almost fifty thousand psychiatric beds. Today, there is less than one-tenth of that number."[18] The reduction in beds would make sense if there was enough care for people elsewhere in the system, but the admirable goal of deinstitutionalization was never backed up with greater care in the community. Instead, people have sought care other ways. The number of emergency mental health visits to the Vancouver General Hospital and St. Paul's Hospital was around 10,000 in 2015, up from 6,520 in 2009. The city's police department has said the number of people it apprehended under the province's Mental Health Act had risen from 2,276 in 2010 to 4,713 in 2015.[19]

According to Statistics Canada, in 2015 nearly 6 percent—about one out of every seventeen people in the country—ranked their mental health as fair or poor. Nearly one out of eight people over the age of twelve, some 3.7 million Canadians, said they had been diagnosed with a mood or anxiety disorder by a health professional. Mood disorders included depression, bipolar disorder, mania and dysthymia, a mild persistent depression. Anxiety disorders included phobia, obsessive-compulsive disorder or a panic disorder. Of those diagnosed with such a disorder, more than one in five reported using illicit drugs within the past year. That was more than double the rate for people who had not been diagnosed with a mood or anxiety disorder. They were also much less likely to work.[20]

Put another way, tent cities are a symptom of a deeper problem. If society were a body, they'd be a fever, a growing sense that something is wrong, that we should be feeling better. They are a sign that we are in crisis, one that is both social and a health crisis. And this, as is often repeated, is in a relatively rich city in a rich province in a rich country. A year or so after officials disbanded Victoria's tent city and found shelter for many who had lived there, it had been replaced with a park including a children's playground. The corner was prettier, but hundreds of people, now dispersed, continued to sleep outside in the city's parks. We'd taken a couple acetaminophen tablets, but stronger medicine was needed.

CHAPTER 6

Self-Medicating

The Overdose Crisis and Untreated Trauma

The number of people dying after taking illegal drugs, a declared public health emergency in British Columbia, is another sign that our society is sick. Midway through British Columbia's provincial election in April 2017, Derek Peach stood up at a town hall–style meeting hosted by NDP leader John Horgan at a Victoria hotel. "We had 914 human beings die last year from drug overdose," said Peach, an older man in a suit jacket who'd waited nearly an hour for his turn to speak. "My child was one of them."

An NDP supporter whose daughter died two months earlier at the age of fifty, Peach wanted to know what his party would do about the ongoing crisis. "Tell me you've got something better than just another phone number or website for people to phone. What have we got in our platform?"

Horgan expressed sympathy. "You and 900 other families are suffering because of a lack of action to address a health care crisis, an addictions crisis in British Columbia." Horgan said he often thinks about the growing number of people dying from drug overdoses. "We need to work together on this," he said. "On addictions, if you present wanting help, you have to have someone there to make sure the hand pulls people in for help. That means treatment beds. It's in our platform."

Horgan also said an NDP government would create a ministry of mental health and addictions so one person in cabinet could focus on the crisis and be accountable for the government's response. "I'll do my level best to make sure those numbers never ever get as high as they were last year," he said. There was strong applause from the friendly crowd, which included Victoria MP Murray Rankin, four incumbent capital region NDP MLAS, other local candidates, campaign workers and a couple of hundred party supporters.

The BC Coroners Service said overdose deaths in the province in 2016 were up 80 percent from the previous year. People between the ages of thirty and forty-nine accounted for half the deaths. Four out of five of them were male. Chief Coroner Lisa Lapointe described the risks as "unmanageable" and warned that fentanyl was being found not just with heroin and other opioids, but also along with cocaine and methamphetamines.

A contact who works in health says the deaths should really be called "poisonings" since the word "overdose" suggests the victim was responsible for taking too much of a substance, an impossibility if that person was provided with a drug that had been adulterated with enough fentanyl, or another unexpected substance, to kill.

Some days the death toll was so bad that there was a scramble to figure out where to put the bodies, Lapointe said. "We have had situations where the Vancouver hospital morgue may be full," Lapointe said at the end of 2016. "So the coroners had to phone around to find potentially one of the funeral homes we can move the remains to, or one of the other local hospitals that we can move the remains to on a temporary basis, until we can free up some space. Which sounds just terrible."[1]

The terrible situation kept getting worse. The spike in deaths in 2017 was far beyond what had been seen previously (see Figure 6.1). Numbers from the BC Coroners Service showed overdose deaths from illicit drugs were up 88 percent in the first half of the year compared to the same period in 2016. In June of 2017 there were 111 deaths in the province from suspected drug overdoses, or 3.7 per day.[2] By the end of September there had already been more deaths in the province than there had been in the entire previous year and preliminary year-end figures showed the number kept rising.

BC was at the forefront of a spreading emergency. In Alberta, the number of fentanyl-related deaths doubled every year between 2011 and 2015. The province's chief medical examiner, Elizabeth Brooks-Lim, said:

Fig 6.1 **Illicit Drug Overdose Deaths and Death Rate per 100,000 Population, British Columbia**

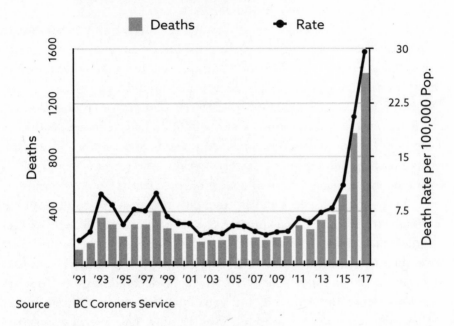

Source   BC Coroners Service

> I just remember nights and nights of going through charts and tables and reading these stories: 20-something-year-old person found in a hotel, 30-something-year-old person found in a basement, 20-something-year-old person had a party the night before ... So it was almost like an overload of story after story after story, and then checking them up against the list of toxicology results and trying to just see the pattern and trend.

By 2016, fentanyl was killing nearly 500 people a year in Alberta.[3] Across the country, according to the Canadian government, there were 2,458 apparent opioid-related deaths in 2016, though it cautioned the number did not include any figures from Quebec and that the numbers from some provinces were out of date or incomplete. In Toronto, where there were 186 opioid-related deaths in 2016, the number of overdose related 9-1-1 calls in October 2017 was up 28 percent from a year earlier.[4] The death rate wasn't as high as BC's, but it was escalating. By population, the rate of deaths was highest in BC and Yukon, followed by Alberta and the Northwest Territories. The west was getting hit the hardest as health officials feared the crisis was moving east.

The Canadian crisis was part of a wider emergency. Opioid misuse had by mid-2017 become one of the most important health problems in the United States, causing nearly as many deaths as smoking does.[5] In 2015, more than 33,000 people died from opioid drug overdoses in the United States, a record, according to the US Centers for Disease Control and Prevention. Montgomery County in Ohio had the most deaths per capita in the country and was headed towards 800 deaths in 2017. The captain of the Montgomery County sheriff's office, Mike Brem, said, "If we stay on this pace, we could quadruple our deaths from last year."[6]

For people living in Victoria's tent city, overdoses were a fact of life, though largely viewed as a known risk. I asked Norm Ruble, who we met earlier, about a resident who died at the end of 2015 at the camp. "That was due to fentanyl and that user being irresponsible," he said. "I say that because he, I can only make assumptions, he decided to shoot up some heroin, had fentanyl with it, and you should never, ever shoot heroin alone. I'm not a heroin user, but even I know that. Even I'm not that stupid." When I asked if the user would have known his drugs included fentanyl, Ruble said "no":

> There's no deliberately mixing fentanyl in with it. It's something it's already pre-mixed with. Whoever sold it used it as a buffer. Not even whoever sold it. It could be from like a bunch of people up the chain just making it extra strong so they can cut it down and buff it up and get a hell of a lot more to make more product ... Just so they make more money. He did not deliberately mix that in. A lot of people had dropped the night before. None had died, but lots had dropped. [They'd] required 9-1-1, or required the Narcan shot.

In the camp, people had access to naloxone, known by the brand name Narcan, which can reverse the effects of overdoses. Ruble said people were looking out for each other and argued that they would be more at risk on their own elsewhere in the city.

The tent city death was unusual. An August 2017 statement from BC's chief coroner Lapointe said 90 percent of overdoses occur indoors, often among people using alone. Often, but not always, people knew they were taking fentanyl. "The majority of the overdose deaths we investigate involve fentanyl, as well as other drugs," the statement said. "Cocaine is often present, as are heroin, methamphetamines, and MDMA (ecstasy). Often, those using drugs are seeking fentanyl. In other situations, users had no idea that the drug they purchased from a supposed reliable source contained this unpredictable substance."[7]

In BC, the effects of the crisis were stretching far beyond the people whose lives were at risk from taking drugs. There were stories of would-be good Samaritans reluctant to provide first aid, worried that they would come in contact with a harmful dose of fentanyl. A conservation group in the Fraser Valley made public that it was cancelling plans to clean up a waterway, fearing that discarded needles could expose staff or volunteers to the drug. Lina Azeez, campaign manager with the Watershed Watch Salmon Society, had bought a naloxone kit to take on clean-ups. "When you start to go down into these natural spaces and see where people are being flushed into, because they have nowhere else to go, they don't have safe injection sites, they don't have supports from the province, it just drives the whole issue so much closer to home," she said. "I start to realize how much more interconnected our environmental and our social issues are."[8]

Which is not to say sympathy is universal. Many are frustrated and some are willing to say so in public. "I shake in disbelief that our governments help addicts with an antidote such as naloxone, only to have first-responders redo the process over and over again," one person wrote in a letter to a Vancouver newspaper. "Addicts should be provided with only one treatment, and upon recovery, given the opportunity to voluntarily enter a 'prison farm' facility for rehabilitation from drug dependency." If the person continued using illicit drugs, they should be cut off from further support, the writer argued. "The addict can then rot in the gutter."[9] While the letter writer's views might seem to be on the fringe, a walk down Hastings Street in Vancouver is enough to suggest that rotting in the gutter is exactly what many people have been left to do.

Others, however, see addiction as much more than an individual problem. Constance Barnes of Vancouver's Overdose Prevention Society has said, "When you've been on drugs for months or years, you're not thinking clearly." Barnes was a former Vancouver Park Board commissioner who had been public about her own recovery from alcohol addiction. "If you're dope-sick and hurting and someone comes along with drugs and says there might be fentanyl in it—they're still going to take it." Addiction is a disease and many of the people struggling with it also have schizophrenia, another mental illness or have suffered from enormous psychological pain, she said. "There isn't anybody out there using drugs who wasn't abused, a victim of incest, raped, uncomfortable for some reason … Heroin will just numb it. You mask it."[10]

Leslie McBain, the founder of the parents' group Moms Stop the Harm, wrote about her son Jordan's 2014 death. "Looking back, with the benefit of hindsight, I can connect the dots that led our happy, outgoing child to become addicted to opioids. Each of those dots represents an opportunity missed, a lesson to be learned," she wrote. "The dots are clear now: the untreated anxiety as a child that led him to self-medicate; the failure of Jordan's physician to find space to consult with and listen to his patient's family; the absence of support for Jordan post-detox, when he was most vulnerable to relapse and, therefore, most at risk of overdose." The danger had since compounded, she wrote. "Today, the increasingly poisonous drug supply is unforgiving. It has rendered addiction and substance use a life-and-death proposition. Every time a substance is consumed, the spectre of death hangs in the air."[11]

After the Victoria town hall meeting, when I asked Horgan what stood out for him from the forum, he said, "What rocked me was to have a parent of somebody who had died. That goes right to your core. I'm so glad he had the opportunity to speak and I'm so glad I was able to give him some hope that there will be a legacy for his child." Horgan said he'd never before met the man, who he hugged as the event closed.

Peach told me he was encouraged by Horgan's response, though the problem is complex and requires a broad approach. "His commitment to have a single ministry with one individual responsible is a big shift.

That's a start." He said he wanted more detail, however. "I was still looking for more specifics. The whole issue for me is so multifaceted, the educational component, the medical component, the justice system." In general, he said, he was looking for "a shift from criminality to considering addiction a health issue," and found that in the NDP platform.

In grappling with the crisis that year, the provincial government had declared a public health emergency and had expanded services including overdose prevention sites, supervised consumption services and the provision of naloxone. It had also funded a joint task force on overdose response with the federal government.

In early 2017, the provincial government announced it would spend money to add treatment beds and more outpatient services. It would also provide medication to treat addictions for people with low incomes. The announcement quoted then health minister Terry Lake saying the overdose crisis was an opportunity. "We are experiencing one of the most tragic health crises of our time," he said. "But in this tragedy is a chance for us to turn a new page on how we help people with addictions. It's crucial that people working to rebuild their lives have a range of affordable, easy-to-access services to support their journey every step of the way."

Canadian officials looked to Portugal, which had decriminalized personal possession for small amounts of drugs and instead offers education and social supports. Justice Minister Jody Wilson-Raybould, Chief Public Health Officer Theresa Tam and then Health Minister Jane Philpott visited the country to learn more about its approach to drugs,[12] which also received positive coverage in Michael Moore's 2015 documentary *Where to Invade Next*. By the end of the summer, however, a spokesperson for Philpott said the government had no plans to decriminalize any hard drugs. "Our government is currently working on the legalization, strict regulation, and restriction of access to cannabis, in order to keep it out of the hands of youth, and profits out of the hands of criminals," *The Globe and Mail* quoted Andrew MacKendrick saying in an emailed statement. "We are not looking to decriminalize or legalize other illicit substances at this time."[13]

Vancouver has a long history of being forward-thinking in its approach to drug overdoses. Along with Montreal it was one of the sites of the North

American Opiate Medication Initiative, known as NAOMI, a clinical trial that provided some 251 participants with heroin as part of their addiction treatment from 2005 to 2008. That was followed by SALOME, or the Study to Assess Long-term Opioid Maintenance Effectiveness, run out of the Providence Crosstown Clinic from 2011 until 2015. The most recent incarnation is the Injectable Opioid Assisted Treatment Program, or IOAT.

The approach from those studies needed to be applied to the fentanyl crisis, said Dean Wilson, a former heroin user who had for decades advocated for greater efforts at harm reduction. Quoted in a series of articles by Jackie Wong that gave prominence to the voices of people who use drugs, Wilson said, "There's nothing wrong with fentanyl. Fentanyl's just another opiate." The problem was that its presence in the illicit drug market is completely unregulated: "The real issue is that we just don't know what's in it, in the drugs we're purchasing." The options were either making it possible for users to test their drugs or giving them drugs made by someone who could guarantee what they contained.[14]

There were also calls for doctors to change their prescribing practices, a sensible-seeming response considering the role using opioids for pain control had played in growing the crisis. As chiropractor Dwight Chapin described the situation, "Opioids have become quick solutions for a growing number of patients with chronic back pain who do not know how or where to turn to get help beyond pain medications."[15]

And it's not just back pain. A friend was sent home after having a hip replaced with a prescription for an opioid that he neither requested nor wanted. By some accounts, the root of the crisis lies in doctors' reliance on opioids to treat chronic pain. In a health care system that's stretched, where doctors are rewarded for the quantity of patients they see rather than the quality of time they spend with them, it can be quicker and easier to write a prescription than it is to find an alternative that may work and to monitor it. Patients who don't want to receive drugs may find there are few if any other options offered.

At the same time, there have been efforts to destigmatize opioid use, to the benefit of the companies that make them. One 2017 study traced the widespread prescribing of opioids back to a 100-word letter published in the *New England Journal of Medicine* in 1980 that's since been cited more than 600 times. The letter claimed that people rarely became addicted to narcotic painkillers, though more recent research has found as many as 10 percent of the millions of people who take painkillers for chronic pain will become addicted.[16]

As director of the BC Centre on Substance Use, a professor of medicine and Canada Research Chair at the University of British Columbia, Evan Wood had been centrally involved in responding to BC's overdose crisis. People question the role of prescription opioids in the overdose epidemic, but the link is there, he has written. "The shenanigans of the pharmaceutical industry in promoting opioid drugs as safe have been clearly exposed and the deadly effects of overprescription in areas where marketing strategies were most intense have also been well documented."

Wood gave the example of West Virginia, which the US Centers for Disease Control and Prevention assessed as having the highest rate of deaths from opioid overdoses. In a six-year period some 800 million hydrocodone and oxycodone pills had been delivered in the state. In Kermit, a town where fewer than 400 people live, a single pharmacy had received more than nine million hydrocodone pills in two years. "Of course, careless dispensing of opioids from pharmacies requires careless prescribing by physicians who have clearly not understood the safety concerns with opioid drugs and the potential for abuses," he wrote. In BC, there was an example of a single patient who had visited 50 physicians and 100 pharmacies to receive over 23,000 oxycodone pills before authorities noticed. The over-prescribing happens despite little evidence that opioids offer much benefit to people, other than people with chronic pain from cancer, he wrote.

While it's necessary to develop a strategy to reduce the prescribing of opioids, doing that alone will increase fatal overdoses, warned Wood. He explained:

> The demand for prescription opioids has ushered in a new era of street opioids, including illicitly manufactured fentanyl. Unlike the relatively bulky heroin, which is derived from the poppy plant and must be surreptitiously imported from places such as Afghanistan, thousands of fentanyl doses can be ordered from China and shipped in a single envelope before being pressed into counterfeit OxyContin pills.

The key then is helping people who are addicted to opioids avoid exposure to drugs that contain fentanyl, Wood wrote. He cited an analysis published in the *British Medical Journal* that found people addicted to opioids who were prescribed a substitute like methadone or buprenorphine were five times less likely to die from an overdose.

"When one understands the harms of prescription opioids for patients who are not addicted and the benefits of opioid [blocking] medications for individuals who have become addicted, the challenge for policy makers is clear," wrote Wood. With opioid prescribing actually expanding in Canada despite the crisis, steps need to be taken to curtail unsafe prescribing practices and thus avoid exposing more people to the medications. At the same time, for people who are already addicted to opioids, there needs to be a "fully functioning" treatment system that includes recovery services for people who are ready for them.[17]

Even for those who are not addicted to opioids, however, there's risk in leaving them to buy drugs illicitly. An illustration came with the mid-July death of Michael Stone, forty-two, a yoga teacher, activist and author who grew up in Toronto's tony Forest Hill neighbourhood and lived on Pender Island, BC. Living with bipolar disorder, Stone had talked about seeking a safe, non-addictive opioid in hopes it would level his moods. After trying to get one prescribed to him and being refused, he bought one on the street in Victoria. He was found unconscious not long after and later died in hospital.[18]

One harm reduction option would be to take a consumer safety approach that allows people to know what's in the drugs they buy illegally. It would mean treating drugs in a way similar to any other potentially risky product, such as food, cars or children's toys. Kenneth Tupper, the director of implementation and partnerships at the BC Centre on Substance Use and an instructor in the School of Population and Public Health at UBC, has suggested doing this by trying drug checking. "Drug-checking refers to a service where individuals are able to anonymously submit samples of street drugs to have them analyzed to determine their chemical constituents," he wrote. Used in some European countries, the practice has never been adopted widely enough in Canada to reduce the risk of death significantly, he said. "The basic concept is to provide information to consumers of street drugs about what is in them. This information may then in turn allow them to make different choices about where, how much, with whom or even whether to use them." People could also avoid dealers who provided low quality or adulterated drugs. And it would also give officials a way to know more about what illegal drugs are circulating.[19] In the fall of 2017 just such a machine, a Fourier-Transform Infrared Spectrometer, was introduced in Vancouver, the first of its kind to be put into use in Canada.

Two BC researchers, Kate Smolina and Kim Rutherford, found that between 2005 and 2012 the number of people prescribed opioids in the province for long-term non-cancer pain had grown by 19 percent, reaching 110,000 residents by 2012. Smolina was the director of the BC Observatory for Population and Public Health at the BC Centre for Disease Control, and Rutherford was a family physician working at Spectrum Health in Vancouver and as a clinical instructor in the department of family practice at the University of British Columbia. "Each year, more people begin taking opioids than those who discontinue, producing an ever-growing dependent population," the pair wrote about their work. "At the heart of the issue is the ongoing demand for these drugs. This demand is fuelled by many factors, including physical pain, psychological pain, psychiatric conditions and/or socioeconomic factors, such as housing, food and job insecurity, and lack of belonging. Many of these factors are interconnected." For example, they wrote, "mental illnesses such as depression are a risk factor for developing opioid abuse, while depression can worsen chronic pain and chronic pain can contribute to depression."[20]

Smolina and Rutherford advocated coordinating interventions across the health care system. That would include providing more alternatives such as physiotherapy to help with pain management, reducing waitlists for patients needing surgery or to consult with a pain specialist, and better access to counselling, detox and addiction treatments. It would also mean broadening the approach to improve public health and reduce the demand for opioids and reliance on them. Like Wood, they warned of the danger of leaving people who are addicted without access to drugs. "We have come to a point where too many patients have developed long-term dependency on prescription opioids. However, reducing opioid availability without providing alternatives may result in some turning to the illicit market to buy drugs."

In its five-year plan for 2017 to 2021, the Vancouver Police Department called for doing more to address the fentanyl crisis and mental health. It's important to address both supply and demand, chief Adam Palmer told *Metro News*. That means both targeting high-level drug traffickers and making sure people get addiction treatment, he said.[21]

After examining the 2016 death of Brandon Juhani Jansen, a BC Coroners Service jury came out with twenty-one recommendations including better access to Suboxone, used as a replacement for opioid drugs, as well as pharmaceutical-grade heroin and hydromorphone (brand name Dilaudid) for chronic users. They also recommended having more and better treatment programs and putting in place better plans when people who are dependent on drugs are released from jail. Jansen, who was from Coquitlam, had died at a substance abuse treatment centre in Powell River.[22]

In a January 2017 opinion piece, then federal health minister Jane Philpott called the opioid overdoses "arguably the greatest public health crisis we face in Canada." She listed steps the government had already taken, including making naloxone more widely available, allowing doctors to use heroin to treat severe cases of addiction, and making it easier to open supervised consumption sites. The government would also continue to work with provinces, drug users and community organizations. Steps included collecting better information to increase understanding of the crisis. Solving the crisis, however, would mean going deeper and doing a better job of addressing the unresolved trauma and other social issues at its source. Philpott wrote:

> We must look to its roots. They are tangled and deep. They branch off in many directions. Prescribing practices and deceptive marketing of opioids are part of the story. But not the whole story. Imported chemicals are implicated, but this is not the whole story, either.
>
> It is true that, for some, addiction starts with physical pain or biochemical risk factors. But for many, the pain that leads to substance use is not as simple as a broken limb or postoperative

wounds. Very often, social isolation and trauma are at the core of problematic substance use. As Dr. Gabor Maté writes: "Hurt is at the centre of all addictive behaviour." That hurt takes many forms: childhood trauma, domestic violence, sexual abuse, abandonment, rejection and more.[23]

Maté, a Vancouver doctor and the author of *In the Realm of Hungry Ghosts: Close Encounters With Addiction,* has said addiction for many people is rooted in their early experiences. Some people, especially those who suffered abuse or other trauma as children, a stage of life when their brains were developing, won't be able to get off drugs completely, he said. "The drug addict is a particular case of somebody who is trying to soothe themselves from the outside because of internal distress and disturbed brain circuits."[24]

The federal government planned to spend $5 billion over a decade to address mental health, Philpott wrote. "We know that untreated mental illness is a common cause of addiction and we need to intervene early," she said. "Addiction is not a crime. Addiction is not a mark of moral failure. It is a health issue. For many, it is a mechanism to manage unbearable pain, an attempt to relieve suffering when life offers few alternatives." Philpott, who worked as a family doctor before entering politics, said addressing those roots requires a society-wide response that rejects denying people care due to stigma and discrimination. "It means building a society where children receive tender attention and adults aren't so isolated and lonely," she wrote. "It means an international search for effective answers and being willing to discuss bold policy alternatives."[25]

Less than a week after Philpott's opinion piece appeared, the mayors of Canada's big cities were pushing at a meeting with Prime Minister Justin Trudeau to make housing part of that response. "This is obviously a national emergency and it needs to be treated like that," Vancouver Mayor Gregor Robertson was quoted saying. "The solutions have to go toward treatment, have to go to health care and housing supports that are essential to ensure people aren't overdosing and dying."[26]

Lawrie McFarlane is a retired civil servant who in the 1990s was BC's deputy health minister. In a March 2017 opinion piece he noted that since 1990 the rate of deaths from suicide, alcoholism and illicit drugs among Canadians between the ages of fifty and fifty-four had soared by 25 percent. Sometimes described as "deaths from despair," it's a key question why they have been increasing. "Stagnating incomes among working-class families might be part of the reason," McFarlane wrote. "So, I suspect, is the age of the population segment we're talking about. Younger people tend to be more resilient. And folks in their sixties have retirement to look forward to. But middle-aged men and women whose lives haven't worked out can be trapped in a darker mentality."[27] Broken marriages, difficulty providing for kids, guilt and self-blame are common, he said. Meanwhile, the supports people enjoyed in the past, such as religion, trade unions or service clubs, have weakened. "You might expect that young people fleeing dysfunctional homes, or kids willing to try whatever concoction comes along, would be the principal victims. But fentanyl is not, primarily, a plague that kills teenagers (or seniors), though there are deaths in both groups." Instead, the majority of drug-overdose deaths in BC were of people between the ages of forty and fifty-nine.

The people who are dying are also predominantly men. McFarlane suggested the over-representation of men could be related to the decline in male-dominated parts of the economy, a drop in the availability of family-supporting jobs in resource extraction, mining and forestry. Gender roles have shifted in recent decades, but expectations that men will be providers largely have not. "The hard truth is, we really don't understand what is going on," he wrote. "The symptoms of death from despair are well-known—opioid fatalities, homelessness, suicide—but we haven't tied down the social malfunction behind them." People point to mental illness, high housing costs, or childhood abuse, which are real but not the whole story, he wrote. "We need a public discussion of this crisis, before it gets worse."

Besides overdoses, men are also more likely to die from workplace accidents, alcoholism and suicide. That's significant, according to Dan Bilsker, an assistant clinical professor at UBC and the co-author of *A Roadmap to Men's Health*. "Both suicide and overdose may be acts of men who have lost hope that life will provide meaning through work, family or loving partnership, men who don't care whether they live or die."[28] In other words, the overdose crisis speaks to widespread loss of hope, particularly for men. The crisis is therefore existential in nature. As

Andre Piver, who worked in the mental health system for twenty years, put it, "Rather than getting high, most people who get into trouble are just trying to get by and stop focusing on worry, hopelessness or just physical pain which, importantly, also may become a substitute focus for existential discomfort. We are in a 'lost' time at the end of this industrialized civilization." Writing from Nelson in BC's southeast, he called for rebuilding the mental health system in a way that allows caregivers to make human connections and build trust with the people they are supposed to be helping.[29]

Even for those working in small communities, the roots of the crisis are not always immediately apparent. Esther Tailfeathers was a family physician and emergency room doctor at the Cardston Hospital who came from the Kainai, or Blood Tribe, reserve in southern Alberta, which was in the midst of its own fentanyl overdose crisis. "Initially, we had thought the main reason for this epidemic in our community was we were seeing the intergenerational trauma from residential schools being resurrected," she has said, adding that turned out not to be the main factor leading young people into addiction. "We're finding out that the number one social determinant for what we're seeing with addictions in this community is poverty," she said. "In order to address our poverty issue, we need to address our self-sustenance … We need to be sustaining our own population with work on-reserve and with agriculture and industry on-reserve that is environmentally friendly [since] we consider the stewardship of the land as important."[30]

After Premier Horgan made Judy Darcy responsible for a new ministry of mental health and addictions, she laid out her thoughts on the issue. A prominent union leader before entering politics, she has said her perspective on the issue is broad. Noting that about half the people who came to her constituency office seeking help were dealing with mental health issues and addictions, she said it had been impossible to know what to suggest.[31] Later, Darcy wrote that the system is fragmented and people wait too long for treatment:

If you break your leg, you know where to go to get the help you need quickly. However, we don't have that same system if you are suffering from mental-health issues or addictions—even though hundreds of thousands of British Columbians are suffering from such illnesses. We need a more effective system that focuses on prevention, early intervention, treatment and recovery—a system where you ask for help once and get help fast.

She continued, "We need to look at underlying issues like stigma, poverty, homelessness and housing, and work with First Nations leaders on the unique issues faced by Indigenous people who are so disproportionately affected by the overdose crisis."[32]

That failure to deal with the underlying causes is long-standing. Diane McIntosh, who teaches in the psychiatry department at the University of British Columbia, has written, "I believe this crisis is due, to a great extent, to the wilful blindness of all levels of government through the inadequate resourcing of mental health care." The cracks that people fall through are the size of the Grand Canyon, she said, blaming the situation on negligence and ignorance, not just among governments and health care providers, but also society at large. Without care, many people with mental illness suffer silently, she wrote. "Untreated mental illness drives addiction and addiction drives mental illness, creating a vicious cycle that too often is broken by death, not recovery."[33]

The overdose crisis, like homelessness and tent cities, is a symptom of a sick society and it speaks to a broader malaise. We live in an economy that depends on consumption and that requires people to need more stuff, to feel unsatisfied with what we already have. Or as a shaman from BC who is known as both Ronin Niwe and Dave has explained, "We don't love ourselves ... That's the root of it. Our society is sick, our society is depressed and mass parts of the population have huge traumas."[34] Or in the words of one letter writer to a Victoria newspaper, "Drug addiction is one of many problematic symptoms seen in our society today due to unfulfilled basic human needs such as love, community and holistic wellness."[35]

That conclusion is similar to those a retired Simon Fraser University psychology professor, Bruce Alexander, has made. Alexander started by studying rats, then extended his observations to people, including the experiences of Indigenous people after European colonizers arrived in western North America in the eighteenth and nineteenth centuries.

The presence of an addictive substance matters less than the social conditions that made people, or rats, want it, he wrote. He concluded that addiction—including addiction to drugs or alcohol, which he described as a relatively minor part of the phenomenon—is more of a social problem than an individual problem, and that when a society fragments, addiction increases dramatically. In a piece available on his website, Alexander wrote:

> When I talk to addicted people, whether they are addicted to alcohol, drugs, gambling, Internet use, sex, or anything else, I encounter human beings who really do not have a viable social or cultural life. They use their addictions as a way of coping with their dislocation: as an escape, a pain killer, or a kind of substitute for a full life. More and more psychologists and psychiatrists are reporting similar observations. Maybe our fragmented, mobile, ever-changing modern society has produced social and cultural isolation in very large numbers of people, even though their cages are invisible!

The flood of addiction that we see is because "our hyperindividualistic, hypercompetitive, frantic, crisis-ridden society makes most people feel [socially] and culturally isolated," he wrote. In this view, addiction to drugs and other pursuits is a temporary relief from widespread, chronic isolation.[36] The problem is not fentanyl, opioids, heroin or alcohol. The problem is modern life. It's a perspective that shifts blame from the person who is addicted to the broader circumstances within which they live.

CHAPTER 7

Healing Traditions

Trauma, Land and Indigenous Health

At a Vancouver City Council meeting in the summer of 2017, Patricia Daly, the chief medical health officer for Vancouver Coastal Health, stressed how much harder the overdose crisis was hitting Indigenous people than anyone else. "Their risk of overdose was 12 times the rate of the rest of the population in Vancouver," said Daly, citing an analysis of emergency room visits between 2012 and 2016.[1] Figures from the First Nations Health Authority, a body unique in Canada that has provided health services and programs in BC since 2013, showed that despite making up just 3.4 percent of the province's population, Indigenous people experienced 14 percent of the overdoses and 10 percent of the deaths.[2] And while 20 percent of all people who overdose are women, among Aboriginals the proportion was much higher at 40 percent.

Grand Chief Doug Kelly, the chair of the First Nations Health Council, offered an explanation to reporters at a press conference in early August 2017. He noted that alcoholism and suicides had been devastating Indigenous communities since long before the latest overdose crisis. "All of those issues have similar causes: It's unresolved trauma, unresolved grief," he said.

> My respected elders have taught me that sometimes physical pain is actually a spiritual pain. Sometimes, a physical pain has a mental cause or an emotional cause. So when we begin to

confront those challenges, we need to make sure that we're responding with the appropriate care: if you need a counsellor, then we need to make sure a counsellor's available; if you need a medicine woman or a medicine man, then that's who we want to make sure we connect you with.

And the FNHA's deputy chief medical health officer, Shannon McDonald, said, "We recognize the root cause of where we are today ... and that root cause rests in colonization, displacement, connection that has been broken." Many First Nations women have been traumatized, she added. "We know that there are unspeakable experiences that young girls and women are having, that—in poverty, and with trauma—people may end up in lifestyles that put them at significant risk."[3, 4]

Perry Bellegarde, the national chief of the Assembly of First Nations, has connected racism and health in his public comments. "Every child has a right to a safe and healthy home and to grow up in a society where they are treated with dignity and respect and have the same opportunities as other children," Bellegarde said at the AFN's annual general meeting in Regina in July 2017. "The violence, the racism, the discrimination has to end."[5]

The risks are reflected in data from Statistics Canada. "The overall violent victimization rate—which includes sexual assault, robbery and physical assault—was 163 incidents per 1,000 people among Aboriginal people in Canada in 2014, more than double the rate among non-Aboriginal people (74 incidents per 1,000 people)," the government agency reported in a 2016 study. Indigenous people experienced higher rates of spousal violence than other Canadians and were three times as likely to have been sexually assaulted. "The study found that the higher victimization rates among Aboriginal people were related to the presence of other risk factors, such as experiencing childhood maltreatment, perceiving social disorder in one's neighbourhood, experiencing homelessness, using drugs, or having fair or poor mental health." Forty percent of Aboriginal people had experienced "some form of childhood physical and/or sexual maltreatment" before they turned fifteen.[6]

For a 2016 report, the office of the Representative for Children and Youth in BC documented 145 incidents of sexualized violence against

121 youth in government care. "A total of 74—or 61 per cent—were Aboriginal girls, despite the fact that Aboriginal girls comprised, on average, only 25 per cent of the total children in care in B.C. during the time period covered by this review," the report said, noting assaults were likely under-reported as some victims likely remained quiet about what they'd experienced. "Female victims in this review who were age 12 or younger at the time of the incident of sexualized violence were four times more likely to be Aboriginal than non-Aboriginal, while girls between the ages of 13 and 18 were twice as likely to be Aboriginal." Nearly 20 percent of the girls included in the review had attempted suicide and half had problematic substance use issues, it said. "More than 70 per cent had at least one diagnosed or suspected mental health issue, with two-thirds having one or more neurodevelopmental disabilities."[7] Across Canada, about half of the children in government care are Indigenous.

In a report for the Canadian Women's Foundation, Manon Lamontagne wrote that the Royal Commission on Aboriginal Peoples had in 1996 found that violence was the most important issue facing Aboriginal communities. While there were "widely varying estimates" of the rate of family violence in these communities, she wrote, "There is a consensus that Aboriginal women are at a higher risk of suffering from some form of violence or abuse than their mainstream counterparts." Community-based studies found much higher rates of violence than government surveys did.[8]

Former community addictions counsellor Bev Lambert pointed to the role of childhood trauma in her son Delbert Davis Lambert's death. After fifteen years struggling with addictions, he died in 2006 at the age of thirty-one, leaving behind three children. "Although I had done my best to help him, and to line him up with other supports and resources, including our traditional Indigenous healers, he could not manage to heal from the trauma he'd experienced in his childhood—the trauma that was the root cause of his addiction," she wrote. Lambert is Cree from the Saulteau First Nations in Moberly Lake and was selected by the Treaty 8 Tribal area chiefs to serve on the First Nations Health Council for northeastern BC. She continued:

My son was the victim of sexual abuse when he was five years old. He was such a loving little boy, full of potential, but the abuse broke his spirit. He shared with me that when he sought treatment for his addictions, and attempted to work through what had happened to him as a little boy, he just could not break free from feelings of shame and trauma. Substance abuse was how he coped; it was a mechanism to protect his broken heart and give some relief to his wounded spirit.

It's a sad, common story, Lambert wrote, adding that the shame the individual and others place on addiction compounds the shame and humiliation the person already feels about the abuse. "My late son was more than his addiction," she wrote. "Sadly, he just got lost. He was not the addict, or the crackhead; he was not the anger or the pain or the broken dreams. Those were just symptoms of the trauma he endured and could not reconcile." Rising out of the crisis would require people sharing their stories, she added. "Our fallen warriors need us to be honest and truthful, so that we can help those who are still fighting."[9]

In Canada, when we are talking about the poorest families and the most vulnerable people, frequently we are talking about Indigenous people. Despite making up less than 3 percent of Metro Vancouver's population, people of First Nations descent were 34 percent of the people who were homeless in March 2017. The chair of the Aboriginal Homelessness Steering Committee, David Wells, observed, "Low income urban Aboriginal people are struggling to survive in an environment where housing is unaffordable and the cost of living continues to climb." Poverty, racism and intergenerational trauma added to the difficulties many Aboriginal people have finding homes, he said.[10]

Chrissy Brett, who has been involved in several protest-oriented tent cities on Vancouver Island, has noted that while Indigenous people make up a shockingly disproportionate part of the homeless population, they are also over-represented in the justice system, foster care and sex work.

People are generally less healthy at each step down the income ladder, as discussed in earlier chapters, but the bottom rungs are where people experience the worst health. According to Dennis Raphael, a York University health policy and management professor in Toronto, the inequities are the result of the market economy and the unwillingness of neoliberal politicians to intervene in it. Race is an "add on" or overlay, he told me, much like class, gender and disability. It's a way of understanding what's happening, but it's not the cause of what's happening.

I asked Shannon McDonald from the First Nations Health Authority a similar question one afternoon at the BC legislature. She was there releasing a report prepared along with the BC Coroners Service that found First Nations people were significantly more likely than others to die from suicides, homicides and accidents, including from vehicle crashes, overdoses, drownings and fires.[11] It was difficult to say how much of the effect was due to people being Indigenous and how much was due to being poor, McDonald said. "They're pretty intertwined. We know that Indigenous populations are over-represented among the lowest economic groups, lowest in terms of educational opportunities, all of these things have played into this, but it's 500 years of history." She compared the people in the report to her own experience. "Myself as an Indigenous person, I'm a physician, mother, grandmother, successful, own a home—you can't necessarily say that my experience and the experience of some of these youths would be the same. I was supported in ways that maybe they weren't." We know that for Indigenous people who have been impacted by personal trauma, we're not providing enough support to enable them to be resilient, McDonald said.

On many measures, Indigenous people experience worse health than other Canadians do. Suicidal thoughts and attempted suicide were more common in 2015 among First Nations people living off-reserve, Métis and Inuit than they were among non-Aboriginals, according to Statistics Canada. Of people in the non-Aboriginal population, 11.7 percent reported having had suicidal thoughts. The figure was 25.4 percent for the Aboriginal people surveyed. Of those, about 42.5 percent had actually made an attempt to kill themselves at some point in their lives, which was significantly higher than the rate among all survey respondents who had at some point contemplated suicide.[12]

Other indicators are similarly shocking. In Nunavut, which is largely Inuit, 61 percent of people over the age of twelve smoke. The territory's cancer death rate in 2016 was twice that of New Brunswick's. People in Quebec's Région du Nunavik were the most likely to die from colorectal cancer and had the second-highest mortality rate from lung cancer.[13]

First Nations people are five times more likely than other Canadians to have tuberculosis, a disease associated with poverty and crowded living. For the Inuit, the disease is fifty times more common than it is for the rest of the population.[14]

Material hardship is part of the story. Statistics Canada reported in early 2017 that 52 percent of Inuit adults over the age of twenty-five who lived in Inuit Nunangat in 2012 had experienced food insecurity in the previous year. Inuit Nunangat is the Inuit homeland in Canada and includes four regions: Nunatsiavut (northern coastal Labrador), Nunavik (northern Quebec), the territory of Nunavut, and the Inuvialuit region of the Northwest Territories. Inuit people living outside of Inuit Nunangat were much less likely to experience food insecurity, with just 14 percent saying that in the previous year they had. Examples Statistics Canada gives of food insecurity include situations where balanced meals are unaffordable, bought food runs out while there's not enough money to buy more, or people in the household skip meals because there's not enough money for food. Women, lone parents and couples with children were all more likely than others to live in homes that were food insecure. They were also more likely to have a chronic health condition such as asthma, arthritis, high blood pressure or diabetes. They tended to describe their physical and mental health as worse than people did who had enough food. "The differences in health outcomes between food secure and food insecure Inuit remained significant even after accounting for age, sex, crowding, education, labour force status and household income differences," the study said.[15]

Ian Mosby from the Dalla Lana School of Public Health at the University of Toronto and Tracey Galloway from U of T's department of anthropology wrote in the *Canadian Medical Association Journal* about the long-term effect of the malnourishment that Indigenous children experienced in Canada's residential schools. "There is sufficient consistency among survivors' accounts to state that, for most of the schools' history, the typical residential school diet was characterized by insufficient caloric intake, minimal protein and fat, severely limited access to fresh fruit and vegetables, and frequent bouts of foodborne infection," they wrote. "It is clear that sustained exposure to caloric restriction, such as that experienced by children at Canada's residential schools, produces a biological complex of height stunting together with metabolic changes that lead to greater risk of obesity and chronic disease."

The effects of not getting enough food—a situation that the Truth and Reconciliation Commission found was deliberate government policy—are passed down through generations, Mosby and Galloway wrote. "Infants born to women whose obesity and diabetes arose through childhood undernutrition are more likely to experience interuterine growth failure, both low and high birth weight and growth faltering, and they are more likely to go on to develop insulin resistance and diabetes as children, youth and young adults," they said. "And these effects are not limited to the second generation: studies [show] the developmental consequences of hunger (elevated body mass index and risk of obesity) in the adult grandchildren of the famine survivors." In other words, people whose grandparents were forced to attend residential schools were suffering the health consequences two generations later. "We can now be fairly certain that the elevated risk of obesity, early-onset insulin resistance and diabetes observed among Indigenous peoples in Canada arises, in part at least, from the prolonged malnutrition experienced by many residential school survivors," wrote Mosby and Galloway. "We need to demand that the next generation of Indigenous children have access to the kinds of plentiful, healthy, seasonal and traditional foods that were denied to their parents and grandparents, as a matter of government policy."[16] Not only should we demand that action and more from the government, in the spirit of reconciliation it has to be acknowledged as a national and societal responsibility.

Helen Knott, twenty-nine years old, is Dane Zaa from the Prophet River First Nation, about four hours north of where she lives in Fort St. John in northern British Columbia. She's a social worker with a master's degree in First Nations studies. For her generation, many struggle to help their older relatives manage their diabetes, she told me, interactions that often result in "them getting mad and then having that discussion around food and them having been food deprived when they were young, and being like, 'I'm going to eat what I want because I wasn't able to.'" It can be a big battle in many families. "My grandma has diabetes too and the other day we went somewhere and she's like, 'I really want ice cream' and she looked so sweet, but I had to be like, 'No Grandma, you're not allowed ice cream,' and I felt so bad."

Knott said her grandma never attended residential school, so the diabetes has other roots. "With my grandma, it was that rapid change of diet, because my grandma went from literally growing up in the bush in nomadic bush camps, to a sedentary lifestyle and then that change of diet." Living in poverty with a small pension, it is difficult for her grandma to afford the gas it takes to get to where the food is growing. When they do go, there are questions about how changes to the environment have affected their food sources, she said:

> Even when we go berry picking, the other year she asked me "are these berries even safe to eat?" and I couldn't say "yes" … We're surrounded by pipelines. Maybe these berries aren't good to eat anymore. Are you poisoning yourself through that process? And watching all the places we used to pick essentially disappear. The one that I picked since I was a little girl and that my mom went to when she was young too, I went back there this year and it's completely gated off because of the pipeline road now. It's a private road. It runs right behind these bushes.

Aside from directly threatening traditional food sources, industrial development drives up the price of everything, she said. "Poverty comes into play with the rise in cost of living expenses, especially when you're living in an oil-and-gas-industry–based town where that cost goes through the roof. Even as somebody who has a degree, it's hard to afford to stay at home."

Across Canada, food prices tend to be higher in remote communities. According to the advocacy group Food Secure Canada, Indigenous people are disporportionately affected by the rising costs of food.[17] They tend to live in the north, where long distances and transportation costs can drive up the price of staples. Media reports describe people spending $300 on a couple bags of groceries, $4.49 for a can of Campbell's soup or $16.79 for a litre of ketchup.[18]

April Charleson, a chief of the Hesquiaht First Nation, described some of the continuing challenges with poverty at an all-candidates meeting at the Hupacasath First Nation's House of Gathering in Port Alberni in 2015. The candidates at the meeting included John Duncan, who at one time had been the Aboriginal Affairs minister in Stephen Harper's cabinet. "We're struggling. We're poor," Charleson said, describing her community on the west coast of Vancouver Island, about an hour by boat northwest from Tofino. The population is spread out and not on the hydro grid. Federal assistance rates were tied to provincial welfare rates that had been frozen since 2007, she said. The few hundred dollars people received each month quickly disappeared when it cost a minimum of $250 to charter a boat to get to a place where groceries were available.

Duncan, who lost in the election to the NDP's Gord Johns, responded to Charleson by saying the amount of help was deliberately set low. "That budget was something that was looked at quite carefully, because we have such a bulge in the population, the youth, the new entrants, the age group that's at the age of being employable," he said. "There was an attempt to basically create a larger incentive for people to actually seek to be part of the workforce where work was available as opposed to staying in a community on social assistance ... That's an admirable goal, and to a large extent it works." The formula doesn't work for Hesquiaht and other places where there is little work, he acknowledged, but said that's a problem for local people, not the federal government, a statement the crowd met with silence.

Despite the challenges many Indigenous communities face in Canada, funding for some basic services is lower than in the rest of the country. That point was driven home in early 2016 when a Canadian Human Rights Tribunal panel found that by providing less money for welfare for the 165,000 First Nations children on reserves and in the Yukon than for other children nationwide, the federal government was discriminating against them. "It is only because of their race and/or national or ethnic origin that they suffer the adverse impacts ... in the provision of child and family services," the decision said in substantiating the complaint from the First Nations Child and Family Caring Society of Canada (FNCFCS) and the Assembly of First Nations. "Furthermore, these adverse impacts perpetuate the historical disadvantage and trauma suffered by Aboriginal people, in particular as a result of the Residential Schools system." The decision added:

> The Panel acknowledges the suffering of those First Nations children and families who are or have been denied an equitable opportunity to remain together or to be reunited in a timely manner. We also recognize those First Nations children and families who are or have been adversely impacted by the Government of Canada's past and current child welfare practices on reserves.[19]

Cindy Blackstock, the executive director of the FNCFCS, a Gitxsan First Nation member and a social worker at McGill University, said in an interview published after the ruling that her organization had worked with the federal government for more than ten years trying to fix the problem. While the federal government requires First Nations on reserves to use provincial laws for specific services, it provides insufficient funding to meet those standards, she said. "Going back decades, the federal government has provided less funding for First Nations children across all those areas: child welfare, health and education." Depending on the region, the shortfall was between 22 and 34 percent, a figure that failed to consider the intergenerational effects of residential schools. "They're providing far fewer services to keep children safely at home for some of the highest-needs children in the country."

Fixing the problem would require supporting communities to look after kids at a grassroots level, Blackstock said. "The other thing is that we need to address poverty. The vast majority of First Nations children go into [government] care because of poverty and poor housing." While seventeen states and the District of Columbia have laws saying a child cannot be removed due to poverty, Canada does not. If a family lacks food, she said, it's a better response to provide food than to remove the child. The lack of options can be deeply frustrating for social workers, not to mention the families they are trying to help.[20]

A year and a half after the tribunal's decision, the complainants continued to fight to have the government make the needed changes. "The federal government has been fighting in court to preserve the status quo," Blackstock wrote in a *Toronto Star* opinion piece co-authored with University of Ottawa law professor Sébastien Grammond. "In fact the tribunal has been so unsatisfied with Canada's implementation of the January 2016 decision that it has issued three non-compliance orders and another is pending." While the federal government had made statements agreeing that First Nations self-governance was critical, it continued to require their child welfare agencies to follow provincial laws that were designed without Indigenous culture in mind, they wrote. Too often, damage to communities had been done in the name of following such provincial laws. "Their application led to the Sixties' Scoop, when large numbers of Indigenous children were removed from their families, thus destructuring many communities and sending the message that Indigenous parents are incapable of properly raising children." While the situation had improved, still half the children in foster care in Canada were Indigenous. "In most cases, non-Indigenous social workers and judges decide what is in the best interests of Indigenous children."[21]

Around the same time, Blackstock was quoted saying she was "profoundly disappointed" by the continued failure following the decision to properly fund First Nations child welfare agencies to address multigenerational trauma and keep more children living in their homes. She said:

> They are not taking action and really obfuscating and making excuses for not taking action. If you listen to the narrative from the government it's all everyone else's fault ... I've seen community-level solutions being put forward to the government that are extremely detailed and well thought out because people have been waiting for this decision for 10 years. They have all the consultation they need with the community, we just need money to do it.

The decision against the government related to the findings of the Truth and Reconciliation Commission and its calls to action, Blackstock said. "On child welfare you can track down reports going back to 1978 showing that the federal government knew about the inequities in family support services and there were solid recommendations to fix it and they didn't.

But these [non-compliance orders] are legal orders and they are still not complying."

Besides more money, First Nations service providers needed flexibility, Blackstock said, giving the example of neglect, which she cited as one of the main reasons First Nations children are over-represented in government care. "I've been a child protection worker myself, so I don't make excuses for parents who choose not to implement change when they have the resources to do it. I'm all about let's hold their feet to the fire because kids have to come first." But for First Nations families, it's often poor housing, poverty and "substance misuse related to the inter-generational harm of residential schools," that lead to neglect. Programs like the Family Unification Program in the United States, which allowed social workers to spend up to $13,000 to help the family of a child who might be taken into care or who was already in care, could make a difference, she said. "What they found was that the social workers were spending it sometimes on first and last months' rent so the families could get social housing, or sometimes to renovate bathrooms for children with disabilities, sometimes to get rid of black mould, or sometimes to buy a washer and dryer for a family with three toddlers. Really, basic, fundamental things." The pilot program kept 7,200 children from going into foster care and saved tens of millions of dollars. "All the good research says that when you stabilize housing, families are much more able and much more successful at handling addictions and mental health issues. They found that 91 per cent of those families had not come back [a year later] to the attention of child welfare." First Nations in Canada have proposed similar programs, but been refused permission, she said. "The structure of the funding in the department now does not allow that kind of innovation to take place at a grassroots level. That has been one of the major pieces we've talked about. You need to increase the amount of money, but you also need to increase the flexibility."[22]

While provincial governments deliver most health care in Canada, on First Nations reserves the responsibility belongs to the Canadian government. When the federal government investigated in 2016 to see how it was doing on First Nations health care, the review showed "the government is aware that it is failing in almost every respect to deliver adequate treatment and medical services to people living on reserves," Gloria Galloway reported in *The Globe and Mail*. "It points to significant gaps for First Nations in primary care, health promotion and prevention, child development, infrastructure, non-insured health benefits and environmental health." Many communities lacked diagnostic equipment and had limited access to health professionals. "Care is not provided outside regular business hours, Health Canada does not pay for palliative care or rehabilitation therapies, a maternal and child health program is not universally available and the shortage of mental wellness services for children that exists across Canada is amplified on reserves," wrote Galloway, noting that there's much more demand for addiction treatment than what is available, just 17 percent of eligible preschoolers find space in the Aboriginal Head Start on Reserve program and there are too few dentists.[23]

The review showed the need to create a real health system on reserves with minimum health standards that are legislated, said Alika Lafontaine from the Indigenous Health Alliance, a collaboration of 150 First Nations across Canada. The government might see doing that as too expensive, he said, but argued the inequity with other communities made it necessary. He asked, "Why do we not ask that question about fiscal feasibility when it comes to a remote community in the mainstream health system?"

Then health minister Jane Philpott was quoted saying the government had budgeted $8.4 billion to improve the socioeconomic conditions of Indigenous people and their communities, including money directly for health care. "We recognize that it will require tremendous effort over many years to close these gaps ... but we remain committed to working with Indigenous leaders and the provinces and territories to do so," she said.[24]

A few months later, in a speech to the Canadian Medical Association's general council meeting in Quebec City in 2017, Philpott said improving Indigenous health was a necessary priority. "Of all the challenges that confront me as federal health minister, the most daunting is the need to address the deplorable gaps in health outcomes faced by First Nations, Inuit and Métis peoples in Canada," Philpott said, according to the text of the speech on the government's website. The current state of Indigenous health in Canada was the direct result of past government policies, including residential schools, she acknowledged. "By a host of measures—life expectancy, chronic diseases such as diabetes, infectious diseases such as tuberculosis, infant mortality rates, suicide rates, mental health issues—it is easily demonstrated that First Nations, Inuit and Métis peoples have suffered from both negligence and systemic discrimination when it comes to healthcare." Housing, employment, education, community infrastructure and other social inequities were causing poor Indigenous health, she said. The government had included $828 million in its 2017 budget to improve the health of Inuit and First Nations communities, she said. "It will provide many opportunities to work with communities to address a wide range of issues—from the fight against diabetes and tuberculosis to the expansion of telemedicine and home care for Aboriginal persons."[25]

Less than a week after Philpott made the speech, Trudeau shuffled his cabinet and made her minister of Indigenous services, a position that included responsibility for health care for First Nations people.

Philpott has in the past been quoted calling British Columbia a leader on Indigenous health in recent years with the creation of the First Nations Health Authority. As part of that process, the *First Nations Health and Well-Being Interim Update* released in 2015 found there'd been progress in some areas, while others had slipped. The report was released jointly from the Office of the Provincial Health Officer of BC and the First Nations Health Authority. It looked at indicators that had been agreed to in 2005 through the Transformative Change Accord: First Nations Health Plan. In its introduction, the report was clear on the roots of the problem:

> Communities have shown great resiliency and many partnerships have been forged as we strive to close the gap in health status between Aboriginal and non-Aboriginal residents. However, Aboriginal people, including those in B.C., still experience a higher incidence of poor health than non-Aboriginal residents as a result of long-term systemic racism (including the Indian residential school system and the Indian reservation system) and its harmful multigenerational impacts on the lives of Aboriginal people.

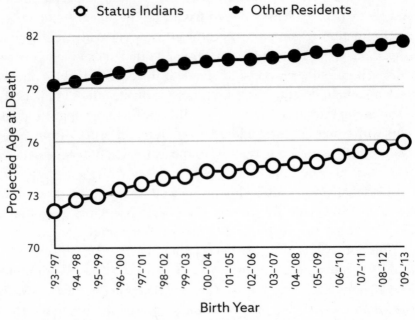

Fig 7.1 **Life Expectancy at Birth, Five-Year Average, Status Indians and Other Residents in BC, 1993–1997 to 2009–2013**

○ Status Indians ● Other Residents

Birth Year

Source   Population Health Surveillance and Epidemiology, BC Ministry of Health, with data from BC Vital Statistics Agency

The update included both good news and bad. For status Indians, a term the report uses for people entitled to receive the provisions of the Indian Act, there had been improvements in life expectancy at birth by 2013 when the data for the report was collected, but there remained a 5.7-year gap with other residents of the province (see Figure 7.1). Diabetes was becoming more prevalent, as it was for the rest of the population, but it was growing at a slower rate than in the past (see Figure 7.2). There had been improvements in the mortality rate from all causes and the youth suicide rate since 2005, but not since an update made two years earlier. The youth suicide rate remained three times higher for status Indians than it was for other British Columbians, the report said. Meanwhile, babies were less likely to survive (see Figure 7.3). "Unfortunately, data also show that the

Fig 7.2 Diabetes, Age-Standardized Prevalence Rate, Status Indians and Other Residents in BC, 1993–2014

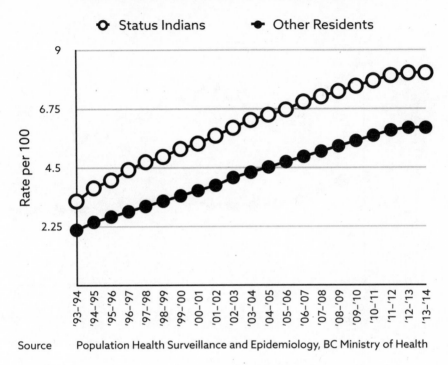

Source — Population Health Surveillance and Epidemiology, BC Ministry of Health

infant mortality rate ... has increased and is currently higher than it was at the last update," the report said.[26] The increase in deaths for status Indian infants happened as the rate continued to decline for other residents.

While there've been some improvements in Indigenous health in BC, in many cases the gap persists because the improvement has been even better for other residents, Provincial Health Officer Perry Kendall said in an interview. And there are promising signs for the future, including improved high school graduation rates and more Indigenous students continuing to post-secondary education. Some communities are doing well economically, engaging in land use negotiations, gaining political clout and a degree of self-determination. Kendall gave the example of Westbank First Nation, which has taken advantage of its location in the Okanagan to open a golf course and a vineyard and winery. Others have a longer way to go.

Fig 7.3   **Infant Mortality Rate, Five-Year Aggregate, Status Indians and Other Residents in BC, 1993–1997 to 2009–2013**

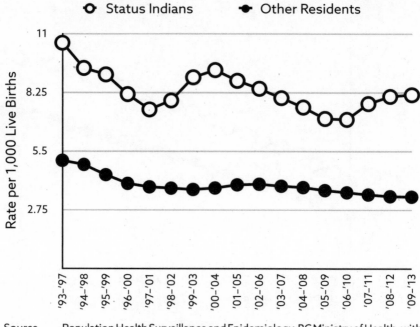

Source   Population Health Surveillance and Epidemiology, BC Ministry of Health, with data from BC Vital Statistics Agency

Kendall recalled looking at Indigenous health around the world for the first report on Indigenous health he worked on in 2001. It was the communities that had more control over their own governance and land base that tended to do best. There are debates about what sort of land ownership is best for Indigenous communities, he said, whether it's better to hold it in common or in a way that allows them to borrow money for development. In BC, First Nations tend to need to go through more hoops to use the land base than others do, he said. "I think it's something that needs to be discussed community by community."

The creation of the First Nations Health Authority makes a difference, giving the 203 communities it serves more control over how money for health is spent. "It doesn't change things overnight, but it's a fundamental piece I think," Kendall said, adding that it can make sure the services are culturally appropriate and delivered respectfully. For example, he said, there've been too many stories about an Indigenous person with diabetes showing up at a hospital only to have the staff assume she or he is drunk.

Culturally appropriate care can also mean recognizing that illness can be the result of factors playing out over the long term. The chief medical officer for the First Nations Health Authority, Evan Adams, has talked about how intergenerational trauma could interfere with people getting or accepting care. "Trauma really is a wound and often trauma is psychic in nature and not physical," he said in a radio interview in early 2017. "It can be an experience that's transmitted through a family over a long period of time. So it can take a long time to manifest and a long time for us to understand." Residential schools would be an example, he said. "I see it quite often in Aboriginal patients in their expectation of how the system is going to work or not work with them." He explained:

> First of all, it changes their expectation and it means that they are mistrustful. It means that even if you are the most amazing doctor or you have the perfect health care system, or you have perfect technology, like a pill that can cure you, they won't receive it because they mistrust you, because their expectation from previous trauma is that this magic bullet is not for them; this health care system is for someone else, that you will give me a colonial experience once again, and I will leave feeling disrespected and with less than what I had instead of a cure.

For the caregiver, that means there's a need to try to understand the entirety of a patient's life experience, Adams said. Many health care workers are good at understanding how somebody's cultural difference affects their experience of treatment, but some are not. "Sometimes it's because workers are not as cosmopolitan as we would like them to be," Adams said. "In a country like Canada, which is a multicultural, pluralistic success story, we should expect our workers to be able to deal with all patients from all different walks of life and all different cultural backgrounds. But sometimes they're not there."

Responding to a question about what reconciliation means in a health care setting, Adams talked about how different people have differing understandings of what the word means:

> The kind of understood, or Western, thought of reconciliation is to make peace with what's come to pass. So for Canadians, it means reconciling the fact that their idea of the country that they grew up with versus the fact that Canada did participate in human rights abuses against First Nations children through residential schools, to integrate those together. That's part of reconciliation. But reconciliation from a First Nations perspective, or how it's been defined by the Truth and Reconciliation Commission, is the establishment of respectful relationships between settlers and First Nations people, or Indigenous people, and a teaching of that past or a recognition that Canada has Indigenous roots. I don't think it's hard for us to do. For many of us it's quite easy and that for others they have to actively learn about it.[27]

For Helen Knott from the Prophet River First Nation, there are close connections between spiritual, mental, emotional and physical health. At the same time, the health of communities depends on how well individuals are doing. There needs to be more awareness of the ways a history of trauma plays out, she said:

> How intergenerational trauma manifests in Indigenous people's lives and how that kind of carries on and that goes into concurrent disorders, so you're looking at addictions, alongside anxiety disorders, and/or depression, which then changes the whole dynamic of family well-being in their ability to maintain health … That not only affects that family, but further affects the community at large.

There are programs available, and she herself does work around violence prevention, but the change needs to come at a basic level, she said. "You can have all these ideas, but if you're just applying band-aids then you're not actually getting to the direct issue of health and well-being, what that looks like at a community grassroots level and what needs to happen at those levels in order for everything to shift."

When I asked Knott what her top priority would be, she said, "I would do land-based healing camps and have those run a couple times throughout the year." Ideally such programs would include payments to the participants, Knott said. "It seems weird to have a stipend for healing or whatever, but because everybody has real lives and real jobs and real families that they're trying to support, being able to do that in that way [would help] ... Everybody has bills to pay and it's incredibly hard." The government's focus has been on creating jobs, but that may not help people heal, she said. "You can create all of these economic benefits, you have that access here within this area, but it's not going to make the people well and sometimes it's not going to make the people well enough to work either," she said. Meanwhile the pace of development does further harm. It's difficult to reconcile oil and gas extraction, the primary industry in northeastern BC, with helping people connect to the land and their identity. Knott explained:

> The economic benefits are kind of railroading what allows people to heal because then you're losing land, you're losing viable land, you're losing animals, that are turning up some of them sick, or having cysts in them and not being edible. When you lose that you're losing that ability to hold onto what you need to create stronger futures.

Intergenerational trauma is closely linked to deep poverty, but the healing requires a lot more than jobs and income, she said. "We're obviously a lot more economically prosperous than the generation before us was, but we're still holding on to a lot of those issues. So I think it's shifted away from the poverty piece, even though I know that's still prevalent in a lot of people's lives, but it's less that and more trauma."

Alan Katz, Jennifer Enns and Kathi Avery Kinew, in the *Canadian Medical Association Journal*, called for a health strategy that goes beyond the provision of health services.[28] Katz and Enns were at the

Manitoba Centre for Health Policy and Kinew worked for the Assembly of Manitoba Chiefs. "A successful First Nations health strategy must be grounded in the principles of self-governance and self-determination, to ensure equitable resource distribution and organizational cohesion," they wrote. It should include support for cultural continuity, language and self-determination, since there is "growing evidence that they promote resiliency and protect against suicide among First Nations youth," they said. "The health strategy should address Indigenous determinants of health."

The way forward will need to be set by Indigenous people themselves. As Katz, Enns and Kinew wrote, "When First Nations communities were asked what it would take to make their people well, they responded overwhelmingly regarding a need to strengthen their own languages and connections to their lands and waters, which have been under assault by Crown governments, institutions and outside society for many generations." The poor health of First Nations people today is the result of generations of policies that also contributed to cultural genocide, they said. "To begin to fully address the health crisis among Canada's First Nations, we need to recognize First Nation peoples as their own best resource, and prioritize the creation of a national strategy that respects and implements a holistic First Nations–focused approach to health."[29]

The foundation is slowly being restored. More than twenty First Nations across Canada have signed self-government agreements with the federal government. The recognition of Nunavut in 1999 created a territory where Inuit people are the majority and where Inuktitut and Inuinnaq are official languages. Several Cree communities in northern Quebec have not been subject to the Indian Act since 1984 and have moved towards regional government. The Nipissing First Nation in Ontario adopted its own constitution in 2014. Speaking in 2015, Ken Watts, the Nuu-chah-nulth Tribal Council vice-president, pointed to some recent positive gains. There was the Tsilhqot'in decision that recognized Aboriginal title, the Truth and Reconciliation Commission process, the Maa-nulth treaty, and the recognition of rights to harvest and sell fish and shellfish, he said. "There's a shift happening in this world where Aboriginal people are taking on greater responsibilities; we're standing up for our rights and Canadians are starting to recognize we play a major part in this country."

Or as Sophie Pierre, chief commissioner of the British Columbia Treaty Commission, said in the wake of the Tsilhqot'in decision, which was the latest in a string of court victories for Indigenous people, First Nations could no longer be second thought. "We're front and centre now." It may take generations, but that renewed standing is bound to result in healthier people.

CHAPTER 8

Environmental Risk
Climate Change, Pollution and Togetherness

The air quality in Victoria, on the shore of the Pacific Ocean and far from any major industrial centre, is normally very good. But as I wrote this in the summer of 2017, with forest fires burning across British Columbia and in the western United States, the sun was a pale red disc through the haze and the visibility was poor. It looked like the apocalypse had begun, a contact in Vancouver joked on the phone. The situation was serious, though, and health officials issued air quality advisories cautioning that fine particulate matter would be at high concentrations for days. In Metro Vancouver and the Fraser Valley, authorities warned of the health risk:

> Persons with chronic underlying medical conditions should postpone strenuous exercise until the advisory is lifted. Exposure is particularly a concern for infants, the elderly and those who have diabetes, and lung or heart disease. If you are experiencing symptoms such as chest discomfort, shortness of breath, coughing or wheezing, follow the advice of your healthcare provider.[1]

The Canadian government's air quality website offered: "Children often breathe through their mouths, allowing polluted air to bypass natural filters in the nose and go straight into their lungs."[2] It was unclear what to do about that, other than worry.

In Kamloops, closer to the fires, the air was even worse. On the Air Quality Health Index, which measures risk on a 10-point scale, Kamloops one day scored a 49.[3] Deputy provincial health officer Bonnie Henry was quoted in the media saying the poor air quality had caused a spike in emergency calls and hospital visits, especially in the Lower Mainland. "Depending on the day and the time of day, the increase can be from 20 per cent to 50 per cent more than we've seen in the past 10 years in the same area," she said.[4]

Similar patterns have been observed during other fires. A 2008 fire that burned 18,000 hectares of forest in North Carolina gave researchers an opportunity to compare the health of people in counties affected by the smoke to that of people in unaffected counties. Emergency room physician John Meredith from East Carolina University summarized the findings:

Those living in counties affected by the plume had a 50 percent increase in the trips to emergency departments from respiratory illness like Chronic Obstructive Pulmonary Disease (COPD), pneumonia and bronchitis while the other counties did not. The smoke also caused a spike in emergency department visits for heart disease not seen in the other counties. People with heart disease are exceptionally sensitive to the particles from wildfires.

Climate change causes higher temperatures and frequent droughts that will increase the number of wildfires worldwide and put both our lungs and our hearts at serious risk, Meredith wrote.[5]

Climate scientists tend to avoid attributing any particular forest fire to climate change, but will say that it's the kind of event we should expect more of as the planet gets warmer. The federal government's Natural Resources Canada website said there are many factors affecting the frequency and behaviour of fires, but acknowledged that variation is "chiefly as a result of the complicated influences of climate change and climate variability." Changes in land use, composition of the forest and the suppression of fires also make a difference, it said.

The department expected more fires in the future. "Fire-prone conditions are predicted to increase across Canada. This could potentially result in a doubling of the amount of area burned by the end of this century, compared with amounts burned in recent decades." Other effects of climate change—such as the increase in the number of trees killed by pine beetles—were expected to further increase the likelihood of fires.[6]

On a warmer planet more fires will also pose a greater health risk to more people. And as with the social causes of illness, it's a risk that is outside the control of individuals and any action to counteract it will have to be taken together.

Besides fires and smoke, climate change brings with it a host of increased health risks, according to the 2017 report of the Medical Society Consortium on Climate and Health (MSCCH). Extreme temperatures, poor outdoor air quality, floods, storms, droughts, diseases carried by mosquitoes and ticks, and contaminated water and food are among the risks. Those risks are not, however, shared equally. "Children, student athletes, pregnant women, the elderly, people with chronic illnesses and allergies, and the poor are more likely to be harmed."[7]

The warning rang true in the late summer of 2017 as Hurricane Harvey dumped a metre of rain on eastern Texas and forced some 30,000 people from their homes. Images of flooding in Houston and stories of rescues dominated the news. Not long after it passed, Hurricane Irma ripped through the Caribbean and was one of the strongest Atlantic storms recorded to date, only to be followed a few days later by Hurricane Maria, another one for the record books.

People who've survived those extreme weather events can suffer from depression, post-traumatic stress reaction and anxiety, the MSCCH report said. There's an increased risk they'll consider or attempt suicide. "Such disasters are also associated with increases in alcohol or drug abuse," the report said. "Beyond the well-known risks specific disasters pose to our mental health, the physical, social, and economic stresses created by climate change all increase our risk of mental health problems."

Hotter days, higher humidity and worse heat waves pose their own risk, the consortium's report said. "Extreme heat can lead to heat-related illness and death from heat stroke and dehydration. It also can make some chronic diseases worse." People who work outside, athletes, those living in cities and people without air conditioning, children and the elderly are at greater risk. So are people with chronic conditions like cardiovascular and respiratory diseases, both of which are associated with poverty. Extreme heat can cause premature birth and the associated poor air quality increases asthma and allergy attacks.

Changing weather patterns are allowing mosquitoes and ticks, which carry and transmit diseases that are serious for humans, to expand their ranges. "Mosquitoes that carry diseases like West Nile virus and dengue fever thrive in conditions that are becoming more common," the MSCCH report said. "Ticks that carry Lyme disease have become more numerous in many areas and have expanded their range northward and westward."

A rise in the number and intensity of heat waves is already inevitable, according to Camilo Mora, an ecologist at the University of Hawaii at Manoa. "If all countries agreed to abide by the Paris [climate] agreement tomorrow, you are still going to have close to 60 per cent of the world's population facing deadly conditions for 20 or more days per year," he has said. That would mean that by the end of the century, the risk would be about double. Any failure to cut emissions will make the problem worse. Or as Mora and his co-authors put it in the study, "An increasing threat to human life from excess heat now seems almost inevitable, but will be greatly aggravated if greenhouse gases are not considerably reduced."[8]

Heat waves are particularly deadly in cooler countries unaccustomed to very hot weather. During a 2009 heat wave in Vancouver there were 130 more deaths than the average for the period. And in Europe, a 2003 heat wave is believed to have led to 70,000 more deaths than normal.[9]

The Canadian Roundtable on the Environment and the Economy estimated that in future decades heat and air pollution could cause 1,200 additional deaths a year in Toronto alone.[10] Globally, research from the Lancet found climate change could cost 500,000 lives a year by 2050, largely due to the reduced availability of food.[11] Climate scientists have been warning for decades that the world's people have a limited amount of time to reduce carbon emissions and avoid the worst effects of global warming. Failure to act will mean many more hazy days, health warnings and early deaths.

Climate change, and the related increase in extreme weather events, is just one way that the physical environment affects people's health. In the summer of 2017, a study came out that exemplified how social and environmental factors can affect not just a population's health, but its very viability. Researchers from the Hebrew University-Hadassah Braun School of Public Health and Community Medicine in Jerusalem had found that over the course of forty years in the United States, Europe, Australia and New Zealand, sperm counts had declined by 50 percent. Sperm count decline had been linked in earlier studies to smoking, stress, obesity and exposure to certain chemicals and pesticides, a report on the study said, quoting researchers who said "measures of sperm quality may reflect the impact of modern living on male health and act as a 'canary in the coal mine' signaling broader health risks." Put another way, the researchers were blaming the drop on both social and environmental factors, which were at least working in parallel if not compounding each other.[12]

In other cases, the environmental causes of illness are direct. Air pollution kills about 7,700 Canadians a year, according to the International Institute for Sustainable Development (IISD).[13] In its report *Costs of Pollution in Canada*, the IISD estimated that the illnesses and premature deaths that air pollution caused cost Canadian families $36 billion in 2015 and the portion of heat waves attributable to climate change—about 50 percent—cost Canadians $1.6 billion. Around the world, the cancer, lung and heart disease that pollution causes prematurely kills seven million people a year. According to the World Health Organization, air pollution was a factor in one out of every eight deaths in 2012, making it the world's largest single environmental health risk. The WHO reported:

> In particular, the new data reveal a stronger link between both indoor and outdoor air pollution exposure and cardiovascular diseases, such as strokes and ischaemic heart disease, as well as between air pollution and cancer. This is in addition to air pollution's role in the development of respiratory diseases, including acute respiratory infections and chronic obstructive pulmonary diseases.

More than half the deaths were related to indoor air quality, particularly among people using wood, coal or dung as their main fuel for cooking. But the WHO attributed about 3.7 million of the deaths to outdoor air pollution. Carlos Dora, the agency's coordinator for public health, environmental and social determinants of health, said, "Excessive air pollution is often a by-product of unsustainable policies in sectors such as transport, energy, waste management and industry." People in low- and middle-income countries in southeast Asia and the western Pacific regions accounted for the majority of the deaths.[14]

Dementia, as well, has been linked to air pollution. In Canada, a study led by Hong Chen from Public Health Ontario and the Institute for Clinical Evaluative Sciences found that people who lived near busy roads were more likely than others to develop dementia. Tracking 6.6 million adults in Ontario between 2001 and 2012, the research published in *The Lancet* found those who lived the whole time near major routes were 12 percent more likely than others to be diagnosed with dementia. The risk was greater the closer a person lived to a busy road, but disappeared for those living more than 200 metres away. In urban areas, about one out of ten cases of Alzheimer's, a form of dementia, could be attributed to living near heavy traffic. It was unclear if the bump was due to air pollution or other negative effects of living near a highway, such as noise. Chen was quoted saying, "Increasing population growth and urbanisation has placed many people close to heavy traffic, and with widespread exposure to traffic and growing rates of dementia, even a modest effect from near-road exposure could pose a large public health burden." A co-author of the study, Ray Copes from Public Health Ontario, was quoted saying air pollution should be considered in planning decisions and building designs to reduce people's exposure. "The real implications are not for individual choice, but at the societal and policy level."[15]

Another study found magnetite particles suspected to come from car engines in the brains of thirty-seven people who suffered from Alzheimer's or other neurodegenerative diseases in Manchester, England, and Mexico. Barbara Maher from Lancaster University said, "The particles we found are strikingly similar to magnetite nanospheres that are abundant in the airborne pollution found in urban settings, especially next to busy roads and which are formed by combustion or frictional heating from vehicle engines or brakes." The finding built on a 2014 study from the United States that found people living in highly polluted areas were 50 percent more likely to suffer cognitive decline.[16]

With the number of people with dementia rising, the reports should give us pause. As an increasing number of people live in cities worldwide, many are coming into contact daily with poor air or particles that can cause harm over the long term. The individual is unlikely to even notice anything is amiss until the symptoms develop years later.

But the risks aren't limited to urban areas. A report out of the Yale School of Public Health should be of interest to the millions of North Americans living near sites where companies are using substances that can cause cancer for hydraulic fracturing, or fracking: "numerous carcinogens involved in the controversial practice of hydraulic fracturing have the potential to contaminate air and water in nearby communities." Fracking involves drilling deep into the earth and releasing a high-pressure mix of water, sand and chemicals that fracture rock and release oil or gas trapped inside. The researchers wrote that their study "suggests that the presence of carcinogens involved in or released by hydraulic fracturing operations has the potential to increase the risk of childhood leukemia." More study was needed to evaluate the risk, they said, noting that for 80 percent of the hundreds of chemicals being used in fracking there was insufficient data to assess whether they could cause cancer.[17]

In a position paper on fracking, the Canadian Association of Physicians for the Environment cited research published in 2011 that found "over 75% of the chemicals used in fracking could result in damage to sensory organs, gastrointestinal tract and respiratory systems. Over 40% could affect the nervous system, immune system, cardiovascular system and kidneys, and 25% could cause cancer and mutations." Another study found an association between some kinds of birth defects and living near fracking wells, they said.[18]

Wherever we live, many of us come into regular contact with pesticides, fire retardants, asbestos and many other harmful materials. But often it is the most vulnerable who are at high risk from pollution. On the Aamjiwnaang First Nation reserve near Sarnia, Ontario's "Chemical Valley," twice as many girls were being born as boys, a trend one study traced back to 1993.[19] Tests by a McGill University professor, Niladri Basu, found mothers and children were being exposed to higher than average levels of pollutants that blocked hormones. Blood, urine and hair samples from forty-three pairs of mothers and children tested higher than average for chemicals like cadmium, possibly mercury and polychlorinated biphenyls or PCBs. There were sixty industrial facilities within 25 kilometres of the reserve in 2013. A survey conducted in 2006 by the community's environment committee found many of the 800 Aamjiwnaang members reported miscarriages, chronic headaches and asthma. Forty percent of those surveyed needed to use an inhaler.[20]

Some 90 percent of the people in Grassy Narrows First Nation in northwestern Ontario suffer from mercury poisoning today, even though the paper mill that released the toxin into the river system closed in 1970. In northern British Columbia, there had been an advisory against eating bull and lake trout from Williston Lake in the Peace Region since the 1980s. The poisoning dates to the 1967 opening of the W.A.C. Bennett dam, which is also blamed for a decline in woodland caribou. BC Hydro has paid millions in compensation to affected First Nations and is on the hook for millions more every year in perpetuity.[21]

In Ontario, as of November 2016, according to a report from the David Suzuki Foundation and the Council of Canadians, there were eighty-one drinking water advisories affecting forty-four First Nations, the most in the country. Of those, sixty-eight were long term.[22] Across the country, 156 advisories affected 110 First Nations.[23] "Many First Nations experience chronic water issues, even when neighbouring municipalities enjoy access to safe, clean and reliable drinking water," the report found. "These challenges are compounded by, and partially a result of, historical injustices First Nations face as a result of the legacy of colonialism, forced relocation, residential schools and systemic racism in Canada." Meanwhile, other traditional foods like moose and salmon were under threat.

Everywhere, people who are poorer are at higher risk of getting sick from environmental causes. A 2011 report from the Canadian Population Health Initiative found that people with lower incomes were both more likely to live near sources of pollution and to be negatively affected by those sources. Over a million people in the poorest areas of Canada's cities lived within a kilometre of a factory or other facility emitting pollution. In the richest areas, a third as many people lived that close to a pollution source. But there were also differences in the impact. The report said:

When examining the rates of hospitalization for residents from the lowest socio-economic areas only, rates of hospitalization for both respiratory and circulatory diseases were found to significantly decrease with increased residential distance from a pollution-emitting facility. A similar decline in hospitalization rates was not found for residents of higher socio-economic areas.

Put another way, poorer people who lived farther from pollution sources were healthier, while there was no such effect in richer areas. The difference "may reflect the fact that residents of lower socioeconomic status areas are more likely to face other health inequities," the report said.[24] Simply put, people who are poor are more vulnerable. Whatever the cause, they are more likely to get sick from it than people who are wealthier.

With the environmental causes of illness, the obvious approach is to prevent exposure to the conditions that make people sick. While there is no cure for dementia, it is often possible to build major roads farther from where people live. There are many cases where the use of chemicals, such as the application of pesticides for purposes that are cosmetic, can be avoided. At times regulation can make a huge difference, as it has with getting lead out of gasoline. Most countries no longer allow the use of asbestos in construction and where it has been used in the past it is treated as a hazardous material.

In making these changes, however, the public interest is often competing with other interests that profit from the status quo and are prepared to use their considerable financial means to defend it. Those interests are abetted by the predominant idea that illness is something to be fixed after it arises, a matter for the health care system, not prevention.

In her 2007 book *The Secret History of the War on Cancer*, epidemiologist Devra Davis illustrated these issues well. She argued that the focus on seeking cures for cancer had blocked what was likely to be more effective action. "To reduce the burden of cancer today, we must prevent it from arising in the first place, and we have to find new ways to keep millions of cancer survivors from relapsing," she wrote. "No matter how efficient we become at treating cancer, we have to tackle those things that cause the disease to occur or recur." Detailing research going back decades, she said acting sooner on the causes of cancer would have made a difference to many. "I believe that if we had acted on what has long been known about the industrial and environmental causes of cancer when this war first began, at least a million and a half lives could have been spared, a huge casualty rate that those who have managed the war on cancer must answer for."

The most famous example of business interests acting to resist action to prevent the causes of cancer is the tobacco industry. It long denied the role its product had in causing lung cancer and resisted attempts to restrict its use. While nobody now would seriously argue against public policies aimed at reducing smoking, Davis pointed out that other industries continue to fight battles that aren't just reminiscent of the fight big tobacco put up but are modelled on it. Industries that produce and profit from chemicals and materials known to cause cancer "continue to use a combination of deceptive advertising, sophisticated scientific spin and strongarm politics" and had remained largely untouched, she said. A real commitment to preventing disease would mean taking them on.[25]

Prevention is central to taking a public health approach. The 2014 National Climate Assessment from the United States that linked climate change to public health expressed why prevention is the way to go:

> Many conditions that are difficult and costly to treat when a patient gets to the doctor could be prevented before they occur at a fraction of the cost. Similarly, many of the larger health impacts associated with climate change can be prevented through early action at significantly lower cost than dealing with them after they occur.[26]

Or in the words of the WHO's Carlos Dora, "In most cases, healthier strategies will also be more economical in the long term due to health-care cost savings as well as climate gains."[27]

The challenge is massive, but so are the consequences of not acting. In a discussion paper on the ecological determinants of health released in May 2015, the Canadian Public Health Association (CPHA) explained the scale of the issue: "There is a growing recognition that the Earth is itself a living system and that the ultimate determinant of human health (and that of all other species) is the health of the Earth's life-supporting systems." There are "goods and services" that people depend on from nature. "Among the most important of these are oxygen, water, food, fuel, various natural resources, detoxifying processes, the ozone layer and a reasonably stable and habitable climate." Population growth, urbanization, development and technological change were among the key forces through which humans were driving changes to how ecosystems function, the paper said. "Underlying and shaping these drivers are societal and cultural values, which for the past 200 to 300 years have emphasized 'progress' or modernization, transforming human societies from rural and agrarian to secular, urban and industrial."[28] It's not just the changes themselves that are a problem, therefore, but the human mindset that gives rise to them.

What it will take to reverse course is similar to the change that's needed to better attend to the social determinants of health. In the words of the CPHA report, to address the ecological determinants of health, "We will need some fundamental shifts in societal values, and with that new principles, and new ways of knowing, measuring and governing." As with the social causes of illness, stabilizing and reversing the environmental causes of illness will require major changes, not just to what we do, but also to how we think.

CHAPTER 9

Healthy Beginnings

Childhood and
Future Hopes

Grand Chief Doug Kelly, chair of the First Nations Health Council and president of the Sto:lo Tribal Council, wrote about the limitations of abstinence as a response to addiction and the overdose crisis. He compared harm reduction policies to unconditional love, arguing that's what people need to help them recover. Supporting someone through addiction is painful, wrote Kelly, who himself stopped drinking at age thirty-four, but found the quitting was only one step and the healing took much longer. You cannot take away someone else's childhood trauma or undo what they experienced, he wrote. "This work must be carried out by my loved one. The best that I can do is to prevent the next generation of my loved ones from experiencing that same trauma."[1]

Kelly's comments reminded me of those from a first responder I heard one day talk about keeping in mind that everyone who overdosed had at one time been somebody's baby. It was how he reminded himself to be compassionate, but it's also a reminder that people who are struggling come from somewhere, and it points the way forward. That hope for the next generation is key. If the addiction and overdose crisis is the result of trauma that children, their parents and their grandparents experienced over decades, then creating the conditions to raise healthier generations will take time and commitment. There's no doubt that what people experience as children, no matter the income of their families, plays out over their lifetimes. Hardship and negative experiences get expressed in poor performance in school, worse job prospects, obesity, diabetes, heart disease and addiction.

Toronto family doctor and author Danielle Martin discussed the importance of childhood in her 2017 book *Better Now: Six Big Ideas to Improve Health Care for all Canadians*. "The children of low-income parents are in worse health than the children of higher income parents," she wrote:

> Differences in the health of children from high- and low-income families begin at birth, continue through life, and lead to differences in health in the children of children born into poverty. These differences are apparent in lower birth weights, higher rates of asthma and mental health conditions, and poorer vision, hearing, speech, and mobility. They're also reflected in levels of exposure to toxic chemicals, such as pollutants like second-hand smoke, and in the rates of accidents and injuries.[2]

Positive experiences, in contrast, lead to better chances in school and work, and to healthier people. Here's what the World Health Organization says in its constitution: "Healthy development of the child is of basic importance; the ability to live harmoniously in a changing total environment is essential to such development."[3] That's true at all levels of the income ladder.

Lori Irwin, Arjumand Siddiqi and Clyde Hertzman prepared a report on early child development for the World Health Organization's Commission on the Social Determinants of Health in 2007. Hertzman, who died suddenly in 2013 at the age of sixty, was a founder of the Human Early Learning Partnership at the University of British Columbia. Irwin is an adjunct professor at the HELP and Siddiqi is on the faculty of the Dalla Lana School of Public Health at the University of Toronto. "What children experience during the early years sets a critical foundation for their entire lifecourse," they wrote. "This is because [early childhood development]—including the physical, social/emotional and language/cognitive domains—strongly influences basic learning, school success, economic participation, social citizenry, and health." The most significant impact on children's development, the researchers wrote, is "the nurturant qualities" of the environments where they grow up, in which they included parents, caregivers, family and the wider community.

But the strength of those environments, the authors noted, depended on wider supports. "In most situations, parents and caregivers cannot provide strong nurturant environments without help from local, regional, national, and international agencies." Investments that support children under the age of eight would pay off over many years, they wrote. "Research now shows that many challenges in adult society—mental health problems, obesity/stunting, heart disease, criminality, competence in literacy and numeracy—have their roots in early childhood."

Children's brains develop rapidly, the authors wrote, so a nurturing environment throughout the early years is of prime importance. They need their nutrition and physical needs met, but also responsive caregivers and opportunities to explore, play and interact. The researchers explained:

A baby is born with billions of brain cells that represent lifelong potential, but, to develop, these brain cells need to connect with each other. The more stimulating the early environment (social interaction), the more positive connections are formed in the brain and the better the child thrives in all aspects of his or her life, in terms of physical development, emotional and social development, and the ability to express themselves and acquire knowledge.

For governments, that means helping parents and other caregivers provide those opportunities. Family friendly policies "that guarantee adequate income for all, maternity benefits, financial support for the ultra-poor, and allow parents and caregivers to effectively balance their time spent at home and work" benefit children, they wrote. Leaders can make a big difference by making sure every family has access to services including high-quality childcare, health care, nutrition, education and other supports. Around the world, societies that invest in children and families during the early years have the highest rates of literacy and numeracy, as well as the best overall health and the least health inequality.

Societies that value and support children and their families tend to benefit, the authors wrote for the WHO. "A healthy start in life gives each child an equal chance to thrive and grow into an adult who makes a positive contribution to the community—economically and socially."[4]

The relationship between a person's brain development during childhood and that person's health throughout their life has been known for some time. "The brain affects the immune system and the immune system affects the brain," Robert Evans at UBC wrote in a 1994 essay with Matthew Hodge and Barry Pless at McGill University in Montreal. While favourable physical and social environments appear to help a person's immunity, the opposite is also true. Lowered defences make it more difficult to cope with what life brings, often leading to depression, sadness and other negative outcomes. Much then depends on the early environment, the authors wrote:

> There are critical stages in the life of the organism in which normal development of the nervous system depends upon the receipt of particular external stimuli or the performance of particular activities. If these are lacking, the "wiring" of the nervous system may take a form different from what it would have been if properly stimulated.

The brain and body develop together, they wrote. "Early advantages and disadvantages are thus self-reinforcing, as they become built into our nervous, immune, and endocrine systems—our selves."[5]

Even from before birth, poverty has an impact. According to figures from Statistics Canada, "mothers in the lowest income quintile were 22% more likely than mothers in the highest quintile to experience [a small for their gestational age] birth."[6] Low birth weight is associated with an increased risk of an infant getting sick or dying, and increased health problems later in life. As a child grows, recent research suggests, physical changes related to poverty can be observed at a young age. "Children from socially and economically disadvantaged families and neighborhoods appear more likely to have thicker carotid artery walls, which in middle-aged and older adults has been associated with higher risk for heart attack and stroke," said a study of children and families in Australia published in the *Journal of the American Heart Association*. Both the neighbourhood and the family had an effect, it found, but the effect of the socioeconomic position of a child's family was stronger.[7] The authors wrote, "Socioeconomic position as early as age 2–3 years was linked to thickness in carotid artery measurements at age 11–12." Risk of cardiovascular disease may begin before a baby is even born, they said. An article on the *Science Daily* website quoted lead author Richard Liu from the Murdoch Children's Research Institute saying, "Reducing social inequality and poverty before birth, as well as in early childhood, is likely to have a significant impact on later cardiovascular disease."[8]

The Centers for Disease Control and Prevention in the United States provides a non-exhaustive list of twenty-one "negative health and well-being outcomes across the life course" that have been shown to rise with the number of adverse childhood experiences a person has. They include depression, liver disease, heart disease and suicide attempts, as well as an increased likelihood of alcoholism, smoking and illicit drug use. Poor academic achievement, poor work performance and financial stress are associated. So is the risk for sexual violence, sexually transmitted diseases, and unintended pregnancies.

Begun in Southern California in the mid-1990s, the CDC-Kaiser Permanente Adverse Childhood Experiences (ACE) Study investigated childhood abuse and neglect and how that related to health and well-being later in people's lives. Some 17,000 people filled out detailed surveys about their experiences in childhood and their current health and behaviours. Adverse experiences asked about in the surveys included violence in the home, parents divorcing, not having enough to eat or a parent being jailed, for example. Most people, about two-thirds of respondents, had at least one adverse experience in childhood. Twenty percent reported three or more. Researchers found that the more kinds of adverse experiences someone had as a child, the more likely they were to have negative health and well-being outcomes throughout their life (see Figure 9.1). The ACE is a measure of childhood stress and its effects are cumulative. According to the CDC's website, there is a clear mechanism stemming from adverse experiences in childhood: disrupted

Fig 9.1   **Adult Health Risks by Adverse Childhood Experience (ACE) Score**

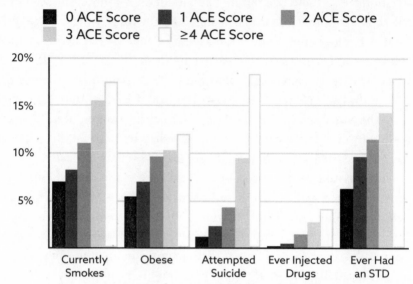

Source   "The Health and Social Impact of Growing Up with Alcohol Abuse and Related Adverse Childhood Experiences: The Human and Economic Costs of the Status Quo" by Robert Anda. National Association for Children of Alcoholics, 2006

neurodevelopment; social, emotional and cognitive impairment; adoption of health-risk behaviours; and disease, disability and social problems (see Figure 9.2). And in the end, an early death.[9]

There are signs we are not, as a society, doing well at raising healthy children. Take obesity, for example. According to Statistics Canada, "The percentage of Canadian children and adults who are overweight or obese has increased steadily over the past 40 years. Currently, almost one-third of children are overweight or obese." Fewer than one out of ten children meet the guideline that they should get at least sixty minutes of at least moderate physical activity each day. "These trends put children at greater risk of developing chronic conditions such as diabetes as well

Fig 9.2   **Mechanisms by Which Adverse Childhood Experiences Influence Health and Well-Being Throughout the Lifespan**

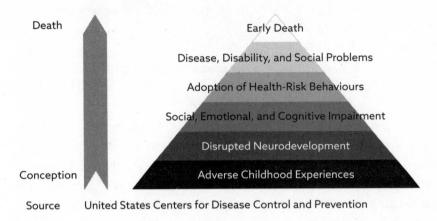

Death

Early Death

Disease, Disability, and Social Problems

Adoption of Health-Risk Behaviours

Social, Emotional, and Cognitive Impairment

Disrupted Neurodevelopment

Conception

Adverse Childhood Experiences

Source   United States Centers for Disease Control and Prevention

as cardiovascular disease and cancer later in life," Statistics Canada's study said.

Data the Canadian Health Measures Survey collected by measuring the activity of parents and children showed that the amount parents exercise and their weight plays a key role in their children's fitness and weight. For every twenty minutes of moderate-to-vigorous physical activity a parent got, their children's activity went up by five to ten minutes. "For every 1,000 steps that a parent walked a day, their child walked 200 to 350 additional steps." Enrolling a child in lessons or team sports also increased their activity. The study found, "Parent and child sedentary time (for example, watching television, playing video games) were also related. Each additional hour of sedentary behaviour by a parent was associated with an 8- to 15-minute increase in the sedentary time of a child."

It's therefore perhaps unsurprising that a parent's body weight also influences the weight of their children. Statistics Canada reported:

Comparisons of the body mass index (BMI) of children and biological parents revealed that a child's weight rose as their parent's weight increased. Specifically, girls were more than twice as likely to be overweight or obese with an overweight parent and more than three times likely to be so with an obese parent compared with girls whose parent was of normal weight. Boys were almost twice as likely to be overweight or obese with an obese parent. These relationships held even after accounting for factors such as child age, their level of physical activity, hours of screen time and fruit and vegetable consumption as well as the age and sex of the parent.

By the year 2030, the statistics agency said, 60 percent of Canadian adults are expected to be overweight or obese, with the rate higher among males than females.[10] And while being overweight can have some protective health benefits and is even associated with slightly longer life-spans, being obese does not.

Among Canadian five-year-olds, only 30 percent were getting enough exercise, according to a 2016 Statistics Canada report.[11] The least active children were in households where incomes and education levels were low. "At ages three and four, children in the lowest income households were significantly less likely than those in the highest income households to meet the physical activity guidelines," it said.

Other studies suggest that overall Canadian children are doing fine compared to their peers in other countries. On a test where participants run back and forth between two lines 20 metres apart, sometimes called a "shuttle run" or a "beep test," Canadian kids had the nineteenth highest score in the world. The fittest kids lived in Tanzania, Iceland, Estonia, Norway and Japan. The least fit were in Mexico. Kids in the United States came forty-seventh. According to *The Globe and Mail*, "The study found a clear relationship between performance on the test and income inequality. The less of a gap there is between rich and poor in a country, the better kids did."[12]

The *National Post* quoted Dan Flanders, a pediatrician at North York General Hospital in a story about a *CMAJ* open report that found 25 percent of eighteen-month-old children were already overweight, obese or at risk of becoming overweight. "It's really not an issue of parents not caring or being lazy. They're just navigating a world where the odds are stacked against them." Cheap, low-nutrition food was readily available, he said. "Imagine how challenging it would be for a single mom who's barely making it to serve fresh steamed vegetables and lean meat and a freshly cut salad," Flanders said. "Our environment isn't designed in a way to make that realistic, and helpful or easy. It makes more sense to stop at the drive-thru and get your kids fed so they stop whining." Stronger social supports for families combined with regulations for how high-fat sugary foods are marketed would help, he said. "Conveying a message to parents that it's their personal responsibility and they need to 'get it together and become better parents' isn't fair."[13]

The Canadian Institute for Health Information (CIHI) in a 2014 report looked at the vulnerability of Canadian children at the age of five, the age when most would be in kindergarten. The measure reflects how children have done in their early years, but also gives an indication of how they are likely to do later in life. The report used the Early Development Instrument (EDI), developed in 1999 at the Offord Centre for Child Studies at McMaster University in Hamilton, which has kindergarten teachers complete a checklist covering five areas of development: 1. Physical Health and Well-Being; 2. Social Competence; 3. Emotional Maturity; 4. Language and Cognitive Development; and 5. Communication Skills and General Knowledge. While the majority of children were doing well on the five indicators the researchers considered, more than one out of four was vulnerable in at least one area, with significant variation by gender and region. Boys were much more likely to be vulnerable than girls. For girls, 19 percent were vulnerable in at least one area of development, while the figure was much higher for boys at 33 percent.

Regionally, at the top and bottom, children in Yukon were more than twice as likely as those in Prince Edward Island to be vulnerable in at least one area (see Figure 9.3). The vulnerability figures for BC, Saskatchewan and Manitoba were above the Canadian average, while Ontario and Quebec were below. Comparing the provinces on various areas of child development, the study found, "Children in Ontario, Manitoba and B.C. had the highest vulnerability rates in the area Communication Skills and General Knowledge. Children in Quebec and the two Atlantic provinces for which data was available (New Brunswick and PEI) had high vulnerability rates for Emotional Maturity, whereas

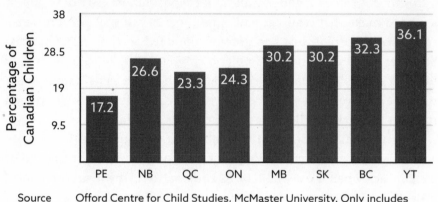

Fig 9.3 **Children Vulnerable in at Least One Area of Development at Age Five, by Province and Territory**

Source   Offord Centre for Child Studies, McMaster University. Only includes participating jurisdictions with data from throughout province or territory

children in Saskatchewan and Yukon had high vulnerability rates for Physical Health and Well-Being."

The CIHI report said that across the country, high vulnerability scores were connected to low incomes (see Figure 9.4). It cited work from the Manitoba Centre for Health Policy that "showed that the odds of EDI vulnerability were 1.7 times greater for children in families on income assistance than for those in families not on income assistance." Reading to children, for example, which has been shown to positively affect development, is less likely to happen in low-income families, it said. While 19.5 percent of children living in high-income neighbourhoods were vulnerable in at least one area, the figure jumped to 34.9 percent in low-income areas.[14]

In Manitoba, the authors of a 2012 report found, "differences in children's potential at school are apparent as early as when they're born and [are] also related to where they live." Children whose mothers were teenagers when they gave birth, whose families were on income assistance or who were in government care were found to be more at risk than other children, the study said. Those living in poorer areas were at greater risk than those in richer areas. "The results show that groups of children facing multiple risks require more attention, and as

Fig 9.4   **Children Vulnerable in at Least One Area of Development at Age Five, by Income Quintile**

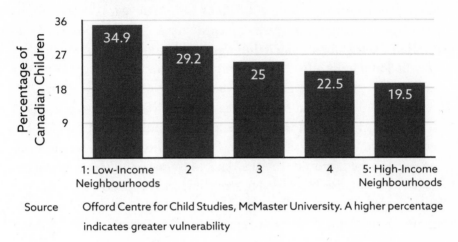

Source   Offord Centre for Child Studies, McMaster University. A higher percentage indicates greater vulnerability

early in life as possible, to get the help they need to succeed at school and later in life."[15]

Exposure to "optimal environments" early in life gives kids the best chance to grow up healthy and happy, the CIHI report said. Meanwhile adverse experiences in childhood lead to a host of negative outcomes that come with a cost to society, including the health system. The report cited research findings that for every dollar spent on programs for young children, society later saves seven. For comparison, spending money on adult education is a break-even proposition. Other researchers have found that not only is early help most likely to be effective, it also increases the likelihood that any later help will work.[16] Supporting families with children better is therefore not only the right thing to do morally, but practical public policy as well.

The results of failing to better support families with children can be tragic. In early 2017, Bernard Richard, British Columbia's Representative for Children and Youth, reported on the death of Alex Gervais. Gervais had been in the care of the province's Ministry of Children and Family Development when he jumped from a window in an Abbotsford Super

8 motel where he had been living. Richard traced Gervais's story over seventy-one pages in *Broken Promises: Alex's Story*: from his birth to two parents who both suffered mental illness, through years of interactions with child protection services in two provinces, to his suicide in 2015 at eighteen. "Constant destabilizing ministry-initiated moves during his early life, along with lost opportunities for him to have found permanence with extended family or a connection to his Métis culture, left him with a burden of trauma that was never addressed," the report said.[17]

"Clearly Alex's death was a tragedy that could have and should have been avoided," Richard said in a news conference. "I do have a greater concern for the hundreds of other kids in the system that are served in exactly the same way." Gervais's story included repeated abuse and a failure to provide care for his mental health issues. "Multiple placements stripped him of attachments and connections that are the basic need and right of every child," the report found. At ten, he moved into the care of an agency under contract to the ministry, which gave the "illusion" of stability, but the social workers who were to care for Gervais tended to ignore him while struggling to cope with others on their caseloads whose needs seemed more urgent. "Left without secure attachments or an education that could have prepared him for some future success, it is unsurprising that Alex turned to substance use," the report said. "His final weeks in care, as he faced aging out with no plan in place and a largely absent 'caregiver,' were a nightmarish combination of heavy substance use coupled with Alex's own overwhelming sense of abandonment."

The report's stated goal was to help prevent other children and youth from experiencing a similar fate. "When a child is taken into care for his own protection, it is the responsibility of government to fulfill the role of the 'prudent parent,'" it said. That means meeting the child's needs for a stable home, nurturing relationships and experiences, enough food, suitable clothing, education, medical care and a meaningful connection to their culture. "In Alex's case, the services he actually received fell far short of the care we expect from any parent in British Columbia," said the report. "Instead, he was left to drift through the care of the provincial Ministry of Children and Family Development, living in 17 different placements and under the watch of a total of 23 different social workers and caregivers after being removed from his birth family. At the very end, Alex was alone."

Had Alex lived until his nineteenth birthday, his aloneness would have been compounded as he aged out of the government's care. The lack of continued support is bad not just for the individuals who age out, but also for society at large, according to Marvin Shaffer, a Simon Fraser University economist. Shaffer was a co-writer of *Opportunities in Transition: An Economic Analysis of Investing in Youth Aging out of Foster Care.* The report found that for every young person who loses support, the government later spends as much as $268,000, a figure that reflects higher health-care costs, greater likelihood of involvement in crime and lost tax revenue from unemployment and underemployment. It doesn't include the costs of homelessness, which affects 45 percent of youth who age out of care, or early parenthood and drug abuse.[18]

Across Canada, the 2011 census found there were 29,590 children under fourteen years old living in government care. Using figures from provinces and territories, Cindy Blackstock, the executive director of the First Nations Child and Family Caring Society, calculated that there were as many as 80,000 children in care and 27,500 of them were members of First Nations.[19]

About 7,000 children are in care in BC at any given time and roughly 1,000 of them age out each year. If 80 percent of nineteen- to twenty-four-year-olds who were formerly in government care received support with housing, food and other basic needs, it would cost about $50 million a year, Shaffer told me. "This isn't a huge amount of resources, in part because it's not a huge population." For many youth who are not in government care, their families continue to support them well past the age of nineteen, in many cases because they make it a priority, he said. "We want to replicate for these youth what families are doing for their children." The BC government frequently says it is doing more than any other jurisdiction in Canada to support youth leaving foster care, but that shouldn't be the standard, he added. "The standard should be what's the basic amount we need to support these youth as they transition to adulthood, and we're still a far cry from that." BC's former representative for children and youth, Mary Ellen Turpel-Lafond, argued for extending the standard age for foster care support to at least twenty-one years old, and in some cases to twenty-four.

Despite the evidence on the importance of childhood and the cost effectiveness of spending money to support children and their families, Canada spends much less in the area than many of its peers do. In a 2017 working paper, International Monetary Fund researchers compared Canada's support for women and families with other Organisation for Economic Co-operation and Development countries. Canada was relatively generous on parental leave, but spent less than other countries on early childhood education and child care policies. "Canada performs poorly in this area compared with other OECD economies," the paper said. "Canada—on average across all provinces—still spends relatively little on early childhood education and child care compared with other advanced economies: only US$82 per child in 2015 (or 0.2 percent of GDP, including in cash and in kind), the lowest among OECD economies."[20] That underspending has persisted for decades and today's results can be understood to stem from earlier austerity.

The thrust of the paper was that by creating policies that support women to work, Canada could improve its productivity and grow its economy. By the authors' calculation, there were 150,000 well-educated women who were out of the labour force while raising children. They noted that the Canada child tax benefit, which paid more to lower-income families, as does the Canada child benefit (CCB) that replaced it, could be a disincentive to work. While the paper was clear on what the authors thought would be best for Canada's economy, it was silent on what might be best for children and their families. Many parents would of course welcome more support to work, while others no doubt appreciate funds, including the CCB, that make staying home a smaller financial sacrifice than it would otherwise be.

David Morley, the president and CEO of UNICEF Canada, has also drawn attention to Canada's poor showing compared to international peers. Among the thirty-five rich nations that make up the OECD, Canada was the twenty-sixth most unequal for children and youth, he said. UNICEF's report *Fairness for Children: Canada's Challenge* had found major gaps in Canada in equity between children in the richest families and those in the poorest. The widest gaps between children were in income inequality and unhealthy eating, and in most areas there had been no improvement in a decade. "One quarter of Canada's kids report daily symptoms of poor health—can't sleep, feeling sick or anxious. This is usually linked to difficulties with peers, at school or at home. Feeling that way on a daily basis interferes with learning, with relationships, with long-term health and risk behaviours like bullying and drug use."[21]

Speaking ahead of an early 2017 visit to Vancouver, Morley said, "Holding up a mirror, here we are in one of the wealthiest cities and wealthiest provinces and wealthiest countries in the world, and yet our children's well-being ranking is so low. And it's a shock." High housing costs in the city and province were connected to other problems for children, he said. "Without secure housing it's really tough .... You want a decent place, and then you can start building a life."[22]

Child poverty has been a persistent problem in Canada in recent decades, a point made each year in annual reports from First Call: BC Child and Youth Advocacy Coalition. "We like to think of ourselves as a caring, civilized society, but in fact we have been tolerating and sustaining shameful levels of child and family poverty for decades," the 2016 report said. Nearly one out of five Canadian children lives in poverty, it said. "By allowing our society's wealth to be concentrated in the hands of fewer and fewer wealthy individuals, we have allowed thousands of children to grow up in poverty that we know hurts their health and ignores their human rights." Stagnating wages, precarious work, gaping holes in the social safety net, and soaring costs for housing, food and other essentials challenge families, it said. "Parents raising their children in poverty are frantically trying to keep their heads above water by working more hours or multiple jobs (if they can), going to the food bank, scrimping on their own nutrition and juggling which bills they can afford to pay each month and still cover their rent. We have ignored the injustice of the continued over-representation of particular populations of children in these dire circumstances." Half of the children being raised by single parents are poor, it said. "Youth are aging out of foster care into deep poverty and disconnection, and a disproportionate number of them are Indigenous," the report said. "Growing income inequality and systemic discrimination based on gender, cultural identity, disability, age and other social status markers frame this picture."[23]

Kerris Cooper and Kitty Stewart, researchers with the Centre for Analysis of Social Exclusion at the London School of Economics, set out to answer the question of how big a factor money is in how children develop. It's a key question, considering factors like parental education likely also play a significant role. They looked at sixty-one studies, two-thirds of which were from the United States. Others were done in the United Kingdom, Norway, Mexico, Sweden, Germany and Australia. Four were at least in part about Canada. They found:

> The studies provide strong evidence that income has causal effects on a wide range of children's outcomes, especially in households on low incomes to begin with. We conclude that reducing income poverty can be expected to have a significant impact on children's environment and on their development.

Put another way, "The weight of the evidence suggested that money in itself does matter for children's outcomes; poorer children have worse outcomes in part because they are poor and not just because of other factors that are associated with low income." Boosting family incomes was, according to the most robust studies, comparable to the effect of spending on school or early education, they wrote. "Increases in household income would not eliminate differences in outcomes between low-income children and others but could be expected to contribute to substantial reductions in those differences."

There are two main theories for why money would make a difference. One, known as the Investment Model, Cooper and Stewart described thus:

> Money affects children's outcomes via parents' ability to invest in goods and services that contribute to healthy child development, such as a home environment that facilitates learning through books, educational toys and a quiet space to study; extracurricular activities and trips out; a healthy diet, sports clubs and good quality housing.

The other theory is known as the Family Stress Model and looks at the "emotional pathways through which money can affect children's outcomes." The researchers wrote:

> Managing with low financial resources can be stressful and have a negative impact on parents' mental health; this then has a negative effect on parenting (for example more harsh discipline) which is detrimental for children's outcomes.

The studies showed, they wrote, that both theories are true: "These theories are not mutually exclusive and indeed we not only found evidence for both these types of mechanisms but also that the pathways are not entirely separate but interact with each other."[24]

Not only do low-income families have a hard time providing what their kids need for healthy development, that lack has emotional consequences for both adults and children that make the problems worse. One of the studies cited by Cooper and Stewart, a 2013 report from the United States,[25] found that families that were allowed to keep more money from other sources without having their public benefits cut were less likely to end up the subject of investigations for child abuse.

Cooper and Stewart cautioned that raising household incomes is not a "magic bullet" that would on its own close the gap between children in poorer families and those in richer ones, but that it would make a difference. "Certainly any strategy that seeks to improve life chances and equalise opportunities for children without turning the tide against growing levels of child poverty is going to face an uphill struggle and place an even greater burden on services that seek to alleviate various negative effects of inadequate family resources."[26]

Another of the studies the researchers considered was by Kevin Milligan at the University of BC and Mark Stabile at the University of Toronto. It looked at the effect of child benefits in Canada on child and family well-being. Since child benefits have been higher in some years than others and vary by province and family type, the authors were able to make comparisons. They looked at how different benefit levels affected test scores, mental health, physical health and deprivation measures. "The findings suggest that child benefit programs had significant positive effects on test scores, maternal health, and mental health, among other measures," Milligan and Stabile wrote. In particular, the level of benefits had stronger effects on the educational outcomes and physical health of boys, and on girls' mental health.[27]

Writing in the *Boston Review* in 2012, University of Chicago economist James Heckman cited a study of what happened within Indigenous families after they were "unexpectedly enriched" when their band opened a casino. "The study showed substantial improvements in baseline measures of disruptive behavior among the children," he wrote, noting the changes in the children resulted from changes in their families. "With more money, parental supervision of children improved, and there was greater parental engagement. In this natural experiment, income improved parenting, but it was the changes in parenting that reduced disruptive behavior." Heckman argued that the key was enhancing environments for children, not giving families money. It's a school of thinking that holds that targeted programs will be cheap and efficient, at least compared to providing broader social supports.[28]

In a response, Mike Rose from the Graduate School of Education and Information Studies at the University of California, Los Angeles wrote that Heckman's article seemed to be typical of attempts to avoid "ideological minefields" in the American debate. He wrote:

> It reflects a troubling increase in policy interventions in poor people's lives that don't address the fact that they are poor. We target their behaviors, beliefs, nutrition, and schools and say less and less about the sources of their poverty: growing inequality, the absence of jobs, lack of affordable housing.[29]

That money makes a difference to the well-being of their children should be no surprise to most parents. In fact a 2016 survey the Angus Reid Institute conducted with Children First Canada found half of parents said a lack of money was hurting their children. About three-quarters of both adults and children said more support was needed for young people in Canada "to safeguard their well-being and fulfill their potential."[30] Put another way, most people understand that while it's impossible to legislate love, forcing parents to provide a stable, nurturing home, you can create the conditions where love will thrive. Money may not always buy happiness, but its lack does bring misery.

Failure to better support families is a significant part of our society's wider problems. Discussing BC's overdose crisis with Perry Kendall, the province's provincial health officer, I asked how he felt the province was doing at addressing the social determinants of health. Poorly, he said, pointing out that BC has a relatively high child poverty rate and that single parents do badly compared to in other provinces—housing affordability is problematic and income assistance and disability payments are among the lowest in the country. Gender, geography and income make a difference, he said, pointing out that a child raised in North Vancouver has a much better chance of being healthy than one from the city's Downtown Eastside or from Bella Bella on the province's central coast. "Health inequalities have been rising, but they've been rising across Canada, so it's not limited to BC," he said. Taking a broader approach to address the social determinants of health would help, Kendall said, but added, "It's largely a very political question."

CHAPTER 10

Treatment

Supporting Incomes and Broad Approaches

When John Horgan's NDP reached a deal with the Green Party to form the government in British Columbia, the agreement included a plan to conduct a basic income pilot project. In discussions of how to better support children, families and others, basic income is an appealing idea. The province would make payments to individuals or households in the trial regardless of whether they were looking for work or meeting any other conditions. The payments would replace existing provincial benefit programs, including income assistance, and could be expanded if they were found to work well. Horgan had told me it was a concept he supported. But it was Green leader Andrew Weaver who championed the idea and campaigned on it. Starting such a program would put the province in the thick of what was becoming an international trend. Ontario had announced that it would launch a pilot project. Quebec, Alberta and Prince Edward Island had also discussed running pilots, while Finland and the Netherlands were both committed to trying the concept on a larger scale in 2017.

Danielle Martin, in her book *Better Now: Six Big Ideas to Improve Health Care for All Canadians*, advocated for a universal basic income that would allow people to cover their needs with dignity. "The biggest disease that needs to be cured in Canada is the disease of poverty," she wrote.[1] Martin is a family physician in Toronto and the vice-president of Medical Affairs and Health System Solutions at Women's College

Hospital. She helped launch Canadian Doctors for Medicare and has been an advocate in both Canada and the United States for universal, single-payer health care. She wrote, "Far more than consumption of medical care, income is the strongest predictor of health. Canadians are more likely to die at an earlier age and suffer more illnesses if they are in a low income bracket, regardless of age, sex, race, and place of residence."

A universal basic income would be a straightforward way to eliminate poverty, Martin wrote. "We can eliminate income poverty by ensuring that no one in Canada has an income below what's needed to achieve a basic standard of living. If we did so, we'd see a considerable improvement in the health of Canadians." Martin cited Evelyn Forget's research at the University of Manitoba on the Mincome program that was tried for five years in the 1970s in the small town of Dauphin, Manitoba.[2] Martin wrote:

> Before Mincome came along, residents of Dauphin were 8.5 percent more likely to be hospitalized than people like them in the neighbouring communities. By the end of the program, this hospitalization gap had completely disappeared. In other words, having access to a guaranteed annual income reduced the likelihood of ending up in hospital by more than 8 percent. This reduction in health care use was in part due to a decline in accidents and injuries. Mental health visits also declined, both in hospital and in family doctors' offices.

There was also an increase in the rate of education and a decrease in health care use across the entire population of Dauphin, wrote Martin. "If we had discovered a drug, a test, or a surgery that reduced hospitalization rates in Canada by 8.5 percent, we'd be trumpeting it from the rooftops and implementing it nationwide immediately."

She pointed out that many Canadians already rely on programs that provide a guaranteed income during particular stages of life, including old age security, the guaranteed income supplement and the Canada child benefit. And when families receive the CCB, contrary to the fears of some social conservatives, their spending on alcohol and tobacco actually declines. "These results are consistent with research showing that alcohol and tobacco consumption may be tied to financial hardship," she said. "Poverty is stressful. Relieve the poverty, and you reduce the stress and its many ill health effects, including the drive to smoke." Poverty also costs the health care system an estimated $7.6 billion a year, so it's worth investing to reduce it, she argued, adding that providing a basic income would be a simple and fair way to do that. "The same principles that led us to establish universal health insurance underpin it: administrative simplicity, risk pooling, reliability, dignity for the recipients, and the belief that access to some basic things should be automatic—a right of citizenship rather than an act of charity."

In BC, Green leader Andrew Weaver proposed a five-year pilot in a few small communities to provide a chance to study how receiving a basic income affects people's lives, the decisions they make and the overall cost. "I think the public would be ready to explore it," he said. Aside from students taking on debt so they can study, a basic income would help people working in what's become known as "the gig economy" or precarious, short-term jobs, Weaver said: "It's clear the nature of work is changing." It would act like an insurance policy, where for most people there would be times when they were in need and received help, balanced with other times where they give back, Weaver said. Pilot projects would allow the government to determine what the program costs and what it saves in other areas, he said, noting that the province pays in many ways for the rising disparity between the rich and the poor, including through higher health care expenses.

A guaranteed income could also buffer the effects of automation, which a Brookfield Institute study in 2017 said could cut the number of jobs in the country by 42 percent within a couple of decades.[3] Many leaders in the tech sector, who see the shift to automation as inevitable, support providing a basic income. One supporter, Microsoft founder Bill Gates, proposes a tax on robots to pay for it, though taxes on high incomes or other economic activity could work equally well. Other advocates suggest it could be paid for with what's saved on the social services it replaces and through reduced strain on health care and other services.

Providing a basic income would give people the opportunity to make different choices about what they do each day. As the economy has grown in Canada in recent decades, well-being has not kept pace, the website for the 2016 report from the Canadian Index of Wellbeing, an initiative out of the University of Waterloo, points out. A universal basic income, offered as part of a broader social safety net, would do more than lift people out of poverty, it said. "It creates opportunity. It provides people with choice. It enriches their lives and their family's lives beyond paying the bills."[4] The arts, athletics and even business would benefit as people would be secure enough to pursue interests that might not be immediately remunerative.

The proposals were gaining interest as people's buying power had become increasingly squeezed in recent years. Reporting on what happened to household incomes between 2005 and 2015, Statistics Canada characterized it as "a decade of significant income growth and economic change." The median total household income—the amount that half made more than and half less—had risen 10.8 percent to $70,336 in 2015.[5] While the income growth was good compared to the two preceding decades, it failed to keep pace with inflation. Over the same period the consumer price index rose 18.3 percent.[6] People might have been making more money, but they were able to afford less with the dollars they earned.

The shift made fertile ground for the federal Liberal Party, which in the 2015 election built its platform around the anxieties of a middle class that was feeling stretched. In BC, Weaver said the remedies the governing party was considering included introducing basic income programs, which delegates to their party conventions had voted for. The commitment could help with a BC pilot, he said. "We would look to the feds to see if they would support it," he said. "It's tough to go it alone as a province on basic income." He also said a basic income program would have to be part of a wider framework that included a housing-first policy, support for child care and a minimum wage that better reflects the cost of living, preferably tailored to different regions of the province. The province would likely be better off overall if it prevents people from sliding into poverty instead of applying the various band-aid programs it does now, he said.

Others have called for boosting incomes to prevent specific illnesses. University of Saskatchewan history professor Erika Dyck wrote, "Individuals with mental disorders are more likely to live on the margins, compounding conditions of illness and disability, creating a vicious cycle of poverty and mental distress." Dyck is the author of a book on the management of mental health. "We know that smoking is linked to illness, and we have anti-smoking campaigns. We know that poverty aggravates our mental health, but we are not investing in anti-poverty strategies. Why is that?" She suggested that a promised increase to government spending on mental health care would fund more services and grow the number of people providing care, but argued "those dollars will not reach the people who need it most." She called instead for investing in "peer supports and client-led governance" so as not to exacerbate the problem. She asked, "Can we boldly admit that investing in anti-poverty strategies is a medically necessary intervention?"[7]

Not everyone is convinced, however, that starting a new universal program to provide a guaranteed annual income is the best option. Peter Hicks, a policy advisor and former assistant deputy minister of Social Development Canada, argued in a report for the C.D. Howe Institute that such a program would be an expensive approach that could take away from more targeted measures to alleviate persistent poverty. New research has shown that "most periods of low income are relatively short, requiring supports that can only be awkwardly met by traditional tax-based GAI designs," he wrote. "As well, for the minority of low-income people who are persistently poor, the best solutions involve integrated mixes of income supports and, often, a variety of services." Better, he wrote, to use technology and data to improve integrated services tailored to individuals and support people through short periods of low income by making access to income supports more flexible. Any guaranteed income program could be used to extend existing measures such as those already provided for children, seniors or people with disabilities. It would be a "bottom-up" approach driven by evidence, Hicks argued. While there's merit in guaranteed income proposals, he concluded, "other approaches to fighting poverty have greater potential and face fewer obstacles to implementation." Those approaches should include, but not be limited to, transfers of money to people in periods when their incomes are low, he said.[8] Elsewhere Hicks called for a new generation of social programs that would be better able to address the complexity of poverty.[9]

It's true there are countless options available. Strengthening income supports for families, seniors and others in need while taking steps to make housing and other necessities more affordable would go a long way towards reducing poverty and making life more comfortable for many. In many cases the programs already exist and only need to be revitalized and expanded. There's an obvious need for more social or non-market housing and for more affordable child care. We should expect that even as we move to a stronger preventative approach, we'll still need restorative programs for people requiring more help.

The tax system could also be tweaked to support people in need and make incomes more equal across the spectrum. Individuals with incomes under the poverty line still pay thousands in income tax in every province; governments could decide people should reach a basic standard of living before they're taxed. For low-income families, some provinces return more in child benefits than they take in taxes, creating significant variety across the country. In Quebec, after it settled with the tax collector, a family of four with $30,000 in income would in 2017 have received $3,047, most of it in child benefits. Similarly, low-income families in Alberta and Ontario receive more in provincial benefits than they pay in tax. But that same family would owe provincial taxes of $420 in British Columbia, $1,672 in Manitoba or $2,418 in Nova Scotia.[10] And when we consider the health gradients that follow income inequities, it's clear that making the tax system more progressive would be a powerful way to close the gap. There's a need to look at whether we are taxing fairly and whether we're doing it in a way that supports families and builds healthy generations.

Part of the needed shift is a rethink of what we value and what we're trying to achieve as a society. There have been various efforts in recent years to measure how well people are living, usually proposed as a replacement for single-minded focus on gross domestic product, which measures economic activity. The problems with reliance on the GDP are many and are well explained elsewhere. I'll just note that the GDP grows when there are more oil spills to clean up, more people in prison or more people who are sick and receiving treatment. That is, it measures as positive much activity that's clearly negative. At the same time it fails to capture much of our activity that really is positive, such as time spent with family or friends, reading to a child or dancing in the living room.

In Canada, the Canadian Index of Wellbeing is the most prominent attempt to broaden what gets measured, and therefore valued. The
researchers use some 200 sources of data, mainly from Statistics Canada,
to calculate sixty-four indicators of well-being. They group them into
eight domains that they describe as interconnected and "of vital importance to our quality of life." They are: community vitality, democratic
engagement, education, environment, healthy populations, leisure and
culture, living standards, and time use. The trend has not been good, the
group's 2016 report found:

> When we compare trends in the wellbeing of Canadians to eco-
> nomic growth in the period from 1994 to 2014, the gap between
> GDP and our wellbeing is massive and it's growing. When
> Canadians go to bed at night, they are not worried about GDP.
> They are worried about stringing together enough hours of part-
> time jobs, rising tuition fees, and affordable housing. They are
> thinking about the last time they got together with friends or
> the next time they can take a vacation. Maybe that's why we are
> getting less sleep than 21 years ago.

On an optimistic note, addressing one area can translate into improvements across several related domains and improve overall well-being,
the report said.[11]

Despite increasing economic activity, in other words, many of us are
feeling more stretched and worse off. Making more money doesn't help
if the price of everything rises even faster than our incomes do and we
lack the time for people and activities that matter to us.

One of the advantages of providing a basic income is that it would be
universal. Programs that are available to everyone are generally simpler
to run and they tend to enjoy broad political support since everyone has
the opportunity to benefit from them. Consider, for example, the general
support for child benefits compared to the stigma many people attach
to welfare payments. The 2015 report *Trends in Income-Related Health
Inequalities in Canada: Summary Report* from the Canadian Institute for

Health Information discussed the pros and cons of targeted programs versus ones that were universal. While universal programs are needed to improve overall population health status, it said, on their own they are unlikely to reduce inequalities and in some situations could even make them worse. The report gave the example of smoking, which for over a decade governments in Canada had invested money in and taken action to reduce. "However, the smoking rate decreased only among richer Canadians, so inequality actually increased over this period," the report said. That is, despite the efforts, poorer people continued to smoke and get sick from it at the same rate as before, even as the rich reduced the amount they smoked.

Targeted programs had a better chance of reducing inequalities since they are aimed at improving the health of vulnerable groups, such as Canadians with low incomes, the report said. At the same time they run the risk of further stigmatizing people who are vulnerable. Also, they would do little to reduce inequalities across the entire income gradient if they were targeted to only people in the lowest income group. "Targeted approaches would be most beneficial in cases where inequalities are large," the CIHI said. "For several indicators, including Smoking, Diabetes, Self-Rated Mental Health, Mental Illness Hospitalization and Alcohol-Attributable Hospitalization, the rates among the lowest-income Canadians were more than twice as high as among the highest-income Canadians." In those cases, targeted interventions could close the gap. "For health determinants that primarily affect lower-income Canadians, such as homelessness, housing adequacy and affordability, and food insecurity, a targeted approach is most effective." Housing first strategies, for example, had been shown to improve the quality of life for people who were homeless while at the same time reducing spending on health, social and justice services.[12] That is, while such programs would not be available to everyone, they are clearly in the wider public interest. They make a big difference in the lives of those most in need, but also reduce the strain on other public services.

At the same time, in most countries universal programs offer more hope of improving the health of a greater number of people. In an interview published on the International Development Research Centre's website, John Frank, the founding scientific director of Canada's Institute of Population and Public Health, said countries like the Nordic ones that have taxed and transferred to flatten social and economic differences have been the most successful at improving the health of seniors, children and people who are socially marginalized. He called for officials writing government budgets to take into account how their decisions would affect people's health. The standard economic thinking needed to be challenged, he said. "Normally, decisions about taxes and transfer payments are made without regard for any public health consequences. They are all made by economists who can't even read the health literature, and with no discussion about the health and functional implications for the population."[13]

When governments make tackling health inequalities a priority, they can be effective. From 1997 to 2010 the United Kingdom's government under the Labour Party adopted a strategy aimed at reducing geographical health inequalities in England. Researchers who published their findings in the *British Medical Journal* (*BMJ*) in 2017 wrote that it was "one of the most ambitious strategies of its kind." The goal was to reduce the gap in life expectancy by at least 10 percent between people in the 20 percent of local authorities with the worst health and deprivation indicators, referred to in the strategy as the Spearhead areas, and the rest of the country. The strategy focused on four areas: supporting families; engaging communities to address deprivation; improving prevention, treatment and care; and tackling the underlying social determinants of health. Across governments, departments made eighty-two commitments fitting with the strategy's themes. By 2007, the researchers wrote, most of those commitments had been met and more than £20 billion (about $40 billion CDN in 2007) had been spent. "Many actions were targeted at areas with high levels of socioeconomic deprivation, including several area based regeneration and health initiatives, and Sure Start children's centres that provided early years child care and education," the *BMJ* paper said. The actions were part of a wider strategy, the researchers wrote. "Overall, this period in England was characterised by a large increase in public spending on social programmes and a focus across governments on widening opportunities for more disadvantaged areas, individuals, and families."

After the 2010 election, the new Conservative government cancelled the strategy. Early results showed that "While inequalities in some determinants of health had improved, including unemployment, child and pensioner poverty, housing quality, and educational attainment, others remained stable or widened, including income inequality, smoking, and obesity." When the Department of Health assessed the strategy in 2010, using data up to 2008, they found the gap in life expectancy between the deprived areas and the rest of the country had widened. "Several commentators therefore concluded that the strategy had not been successful," the BMJ report said. That conclusion may, however, have been premature. Taking another look, the researchers suggested the effects of the strategy took time to play out and that the earlier assessment had failed to look at how the trend on health inequalities had shifted.

Updated data for life expectancy became available in 2011 and data wasn't available for the full strategy period until 2013, giving the later researchers a fuller view of what had happened. They compared health results from before (1983–2003), during (2004–12) and after (2013–15) the period when the strategy was in place. Focusing on life expectancy at birth in the "most deprived local authorities in England" and the rest of the country, the researchers found that the gap declined while the strategy was in place. This stood in contrast to the periods before and after, during which the gap increased. "By 2012 the gap in male life expectancy was 1.2 years smaller ... and the gap in female life expectancy was 0.6 years smaller ... than it would have been if the trends in inequalities before the strategy had continued," the researchers wrote.

After reassessing, the researchers concluded that the English health inequalities strategy had in fact succeeded. Geographical health inequalities had decreased during the period, including for life expectancy, reversing a long-term trend. Pursuing similar strategies in the future with social investments targeted at the most deprived parts of the country could be expected to be effective, they wrote. Not only that, but after the strategy ended, the trend reverted to where it had been before the strategy was implemented. "Inequalities have started to increase again," they wrote. "The concerns are that current policies are reversing the achievements of the strategy." The government, under Prime Minister Theresa May, had said it wanted to reduce health inequities, but was instead pursuing policies that risked widening the gap, they wrote.[14]

The United Kingdom's experience was not unique. Journalist Crawford Kilian quoted *The Body Economic: Why Austerity Kills* by David Stuckler and Sanjay Basu on the effects of the New Deal in the United States after Franklin Delano Roosevelt's 1933 election:

> The New Deal had a momentous effect on the public's health. Although it was not designed with public health in mind, its support meant the difference between losing healthcare and keeping it; between going hungry and having enough food on the table; between homelessness and having a roof overhead. In providing indirect support to maintain people's well-being, the New Deal was in effect the biggest public health program ever to have been implemented in the United States.

For every $100 per person spent under the program, there were eighteen fewer deaths from pneumonia and four fewer suicides per 100,000 people, the authors found. There were also eighteen fewer infant deaths per 1,000 live births.

Another "natural experiment" happened in the 1990s with the fall of communism, the breakup of the Soviet Union, rapid privatization of the country's economy and massive job losses. "The rate of death rose by a disconcerting 90 per cent among the subgroup of men aged twenty-five to thirty-nine, in the prime of their lives," Stuckler and Basu wrote. The deaths were largely from alcohol poisonings, suicides, homicides, injuries and heart attacks. In other words, they were from the effects of stress. "Across Russia ... alcohol was estimated to have accounted for at least two of every five deaths among Russian working-age men during the 1990s, totaling 4 million deaths across the former Soviet Union."[15] The experiences from Russia, the United States and the United Kingdom all point in the same direction: whether creating social upheaval or providing support, government policies have a far-reaching impact on people's health.

In *Social Determinants of Health: The Canadian Facts*, Juha Mikkonen and Dennis Raphael quoted the World Health Organization saying that "health damaging experiences" are the result of "a toxic combination of poor social policies and programmes, unfair economic arrangements, and bad politics." In Canada, people are generally healthier than Americans, our closest neighbours, but compared to people living in countries that have chosen to develop public policies aimed at strengthening the social determinants of health we are unhealthier, wrote Mikkonen and Raphael. They continued:

> There has been little effort by Canadian governments and policy-makers to improve the social determinants of health through public policy action. Canada compares unfavourably to other wealthy developed nations in its support of citizens as they navigate the life span. Our income inequality and poverty rates are growing and are among the highest of wealthy developed nations. Canadian spending in support of families, persons with disabilities, older Canadians, and employment training is also among the lowest of these same wealthy developed nations.

Better public policies for Canada are entirely possible, they wrote. "They have been implemented in many wealthy industrialized nations—most of which are not as wealthy as Canada—to good effect." In fact, they are part of our own tradition as well, though Mikkonen and Raphael stretch back to the great Depression and the years after World War II for examples that include medicare, public pensions, unemployment insurance and affordable housing programs. "Canada has strayed from this tradition and has come to be a social determinants of health laggard among wealthy developed nations. Governments at all levels have neglected the factors necessary for health." Politicians seem to be aware, but are failing to act, they wrote. "Social and political movements must be developed that will pressure governments and policymakers to enact health-supporting public policy."[16]

In recent decades much has been learned about the health inequities that arise from social inequities. Few would now dispute the importance of early childhood, when brains are developing, in determining how a person will do in school and later in life. But it seems that the more is known, the less interest there is in acting on the knowledge, even as generations of politicians have piled up reports on the topic.

CHAPTER 11

Prevention

Persistent Blockages and Sunny Ways

In August 2017, after nearly two years as health minister, Jane Philpott addressed the Canadian Medical Association's general council meeting in Quebec City and called on doctors to advocate for social change. "Here's my bottom line," Philpott said, according to the text of the speech published on the government's website. "For Canada to thrive, we need to improve the health of our most vulnerable people. To do so successfully, we need Canada's doctors to be actively engaged in population health." She continued, echoing the advice she'd given a daughter starting medical school (see Chapter 1):

> We entered medical school with a desire to serve people in need, to improve people's health. Most doctors see this as our top priority—providing high quality care for individual patients. Curiously, when it comes to the health of the population as a whole, it is not entirely clear what role doctors have. What obligation do we bear toward people who don't find their way into our clinics or hospitals or who don't get there soon enough? Who is responsible for the health of vulnerable populations? If not doctors, is it hospitals, regional health authorities, public health departments, governments, or patients themselves? Surely improving population health is a shared responsibility.

Philpott focused her comments on Indigenous health, the epidemic of opioid overdose deaths and youth mental wellness, which she described as linked to each other and to the social determinants of health. "I do not believe that we can achieve a healthy population without the expertise and active engagement of Canada's doctors," Philpott said. "Of course doctors can't address the needs of vulnerable people without a broad range of other health professionals and social systems. But those systems will not succeed without the participation of physicians." Doctors care and they have education, insight and practical wisdom, she said. "Because you are a doctor, society has granted you power and privilege, respect and responsibility. There is no better use of that power, than to advocate on behalf of those who do not have the same opportunities."[1]

While the speech sounded great and identified several areas where the government was spending money to deal with crises, it fell far short of committing the government to a wide-ranging plan to make Canadian society more equal. Instead of really taking broad action, Philpott was calling on doctors in the audience at the CMA meeting to advocate for action. It was an all the more ironic tack to take considering the organization had itself been pressing for more action from governments since at least 2012. Here's the CMA's official position from its website:

> The CMA believes the social determinants of health can have a larger impact on individual and population health than the health care system. The CMA also believes that any actions to improve health and tackle health inequity must address the social determinants and their impact on daily life.[2]

In 2013 the CMA led a national dialogue with town hall meetings in cities across the country. "In those town hall meetings, Canadians served notice that they expect government action to address these issues," the website said. The resulting report, *Health Care in Canada: What Makes Us Sick?* included the conclusion that "Canadian society has suffered from a lack of imagination, will and leadership to address social inequities." While there is a role for citizens, physicians and communities to help deal with the problems, it said, "Governments need to be pressured to take action." Out of a dozen recommendations in the report, eight were explicitly for federal, provincial or territorial governments. The other four included adopting a housing first strategy to deal with homelessness, developing a national food security program and other initiatives that would at least require government leadership, if not direct government management.[3]

In short, the CMA had committed to pressing the government for action and had been rewarded, four years later, with a speech from the minister in charge telling them they had to advocate. The river of rhetoric was starting to look more like a lazily turning whirlpool.

In the time I worked on this book, Philpott was unavailable to me for an interview. Communications staff took the requests I made over six months, said the minister would likely want to talk about the topic, but never followed through to make her available. Less than a week after Philpott delivered her speech to the CMA, Prime Minister Justin Trudeau shuffled her out of health and made her the minister of Indigenous services, a position that included responsibility for health care for First Nations people living on reserves, a job where some observers said she would be well positioned to address the social determinants of health. Maybe this time it will come true.

When I asked Roy Romanow in the summer of 2017 how Canada had done at addressing the social determinants of health, he said, simply, "I would say we have been unsuccessful overall."

Romanow was the premier of Saskatchewan from 1991 to 2001 and the head of a Royal Commission on the Future of Healthcare in Canada that in 2002 submitted to the House of Commons its report *Building on Values: The Future of Health Care in Canada*. The report received some criticism[4] for paying insufficient attention to the social determinants of health, but Romanow says it was produced in eighteen months with a limited mandate. The focus was on how to fix the health care system, not how to make Canadians healthier, which is another question. Since that time Romanow has worked with the Atkinson Foundation and other groups to more directly address the underlying causes of illness. By his estimation he at one point was giving twenty speeches a year on the topic. "I had the impression there was a generally accepted message," he said. And yet, he added, "Nothing ever happened." That could be dispiriting, he said. "It's a very, very tough field in which to labour, I've found ... I'm not sure I've got the will to keep pounding away at it."

In a paper for the journal *Health Promotion International*, Dennis Raphael from York University and Ph.D. student Ambreen Sayani also expressed frustration with the lack of progress. They wrote:

> What has emerged is a bewildering situation in which Canadian researchers, funded by federal and provincial agencies, carry out [social determinants of health]-related research ... and public health authorities recognize their importance in statements and documents, yet little public policy activity specifically designed to address [social determinants of health] is seen.

Citing Fran Baum's work, they said getting officials to use public policy to work towards health equity would require both commitment from governments and pressure from civil society. "Not only is top-down political will lacking in Canada, the Canadian public is largely unaware of these issues, suggesting a profound need for public education and mobilization," they wrote.[5]

Speaking on the phone, Raphael said he was feeling pessimistic about the commitment of politicians to acting on the social determinants of health. "There's a much greater awareness of all this, but none of this has percolated to any level of government, to any public policies. It doesn't get onto the public policy agenda. It's not part of the public debate." He was particularly critical of the four candidates in the federal NDP's leadership race underway at the time, none of whom he felt was taking the issue on. "We're handing them an issue on a plate that says social democracy is good for heart disease," he said. Child poverty causes heart disease, diabetes and arthritis, he said. "How can this not be compelling? But it's not, to date."

Asked why he was focusing his frustration on the NDP, Raphael said, "I have no expectation that the Liberals are going to do anything." Trudeau's Liberals were unlikely to make the deep structural changes that were needed, he said. "I don't expect Trudeau to take us seriously.

I don't expect the Conservatives ... The powers that be, the system is working very well for them. The system works really well for Trudeau. It works really well for these people." When you start talking about how wages and housing affect people's health, he said, "You begin to run into entrenched interests." Banks and other businesses resist change on those fronts, he said, so Trudeau and the Liberals were unlikely to force it:

> They'll do everything they can to divert us from the fact public policy is creating unfavourable living and working conditions that create diseases. They do that because people are profiting from it ... Inequality, poverty, is profitable. It's profitable for the banks, Walmart. If it wasn't profitable, we'd get rid of it tomorrow.

It's easier for a politician or a public health advocate to tell people to get some exercise and eat their fruits and vegetables than it is to advocate for restructuring our economy, raising wages and improving working conditions, he said.

A big part of the battle is philosophical, meaning it has to do with how we view ourselves and the story we tell about what it is we're trying to achieve as a society. "In North America we're embedded in the trough of neoliberal ideology," Raphael explained. The narrative around individualism and lifestyle is so strong that it's difficult to get anyone to take the broader determinants of health seriously, he said. The problem extends to economic inequality, which tends to be exacerbated by governments. Despite home prices ballooning to the point where many people are priced out of the market, he said, "If housing prices stabilize, that's seen as a problem." Economic growth, business success, the market and efficiency are given priority over everything else, he said. "I think it comes down to unwillingness to intervene in the market economy."

Politicians have unquestionably been attentive to the wishes of the corporate interests that have funded political parties and sent lobbyists to make their views known. At the same time, in a democracy, a great deal of calculation goes into figuring out what the public wants or will at least tolerate. Whether through polling or instinct, successful politicians seem able to aggregate that public opinion, discerning whether the moment calls for promises of deficit-financed social spending or renewed austerity.

According to Roy Romanow, the former NDP premier of Saskatchewan, the main challenge for politicians is the prevalent and mistaken view that providing robust social services isn't really about health. "The faith in hard medicine is pretty strong," Romanow said. "I think it comes down to the attraction that we're steadily making progress on the illness side of things." When Canadians talk about "health," the perception is that what's really important is having the latest technology or a sufficient number of hospital beds, and that drives the decisions politicians make on their behalf. Many people, he said, seem to think "you can live any way you want—smoke, drink, whatever you want—given proper money the downstream will look after you." People seem to believe that even if the health care system can't cure you, it's a failure and it really *should* be able to, he said.

The media contributes, said Romanow, with the latest advances given glowing attention on newscasts and in newspapers. "It is exciting news to hear there's a possibility of a breakthrough," he said. With the public attention there, that's what gets the attention of the policy makers, he said, adding there are more political points to score for the politician who announces an addition for the local hospital than there are for giving any number of speeches on early childhood development or prenatal care. "That's my assessment as a former politician."

Romanow compared the policy options to a teeter-totter, with acute care at one end and the social determinants of health at the other. "We still seem to be focused on the acute care end of the teeter-totter," he said. Other countries—Britain, France, Sweden and the other Nordic countries—get the balance better, he said. The United States, with the highest health care costs and the worst outcomes, gets it worse. "It's always the balance. There's never enough money to go around."

Advocates in North America tend to see northern Europe as being far ahead on these questions. There is a stronger cultural emphasis on supporting each other and greater acceptance of the idea that social spending will lead to a healthier population. But there are challenges there as well, as a group of researchers writing for EuroHealthNet concluded. "Many barriers hamper advocacy for health equity, including the contemporary economic zeitgeist, the biomedical health perspective, and difficulties cooperating across policy sectors on the issue," they wrote. That created room for advocacy organizations to take on a central role to bridge civil society, researchers and public policy. "Effective advocacy should include persistent efforts to raise awareness and understanding of the social determinants of health. Education on the social determinants as part of medical training should be encouraged, including professional training within disadvantaged communities."[6] In Europe as in Canada, getting the balance right is a matter of constant negotiation.

Another former politician, Tom Perry, entered British Columbia provincial politics from medicine, experience that had given him a strong understanding of what it is that contributes to people's health. He said he remembers learning in medical school classes the importance of the social determinants of health and the relatively minor role medicine plays. "You then rapidly forgot it because no, we're good, we're the heroes, the saviours," he said on the phone from his vacation home in New Denver, BC. Perry was an MLA for just over seven years and for about twenty-two months in the early 1990s was in the cabinet, serving as the minister for advanced education, training and technology. Many of his cabinet colleagues—including then premier Mike Harcourt—had an understanding of the social determinants of health and a desire to do something to address them, but it was always a challenge, he said.

Perry recalled contract awards to health care unions trumping other spending options. Addressing the social determinants of health was a lesser priority. "It just can't compete really against powerful people," he said. "You can understand it, yet there's no constituency for it." People who are really poor don't vote and the small number of activists who care about the issue are likely so committed that they would be critical of all the parties on the issue, including the NDP, he said. "They're probably concentrated in a very small number of ridings ... It certainly never figured in my campaigns." He later added, "The biggest thing is there's no effective constituency."

There is, however, a block of people committed to keeping things the way they are, including the many people who've built careers on it. "We're all feeding off this carcass," Perry said. "I don't think it's ever discussed, we need the disease care system to make a living." Medical advances that save lives that in the past would likely have been lost lead to the survival of people with ongoing needs for care. That's good for the health care system and the people who work in it, but bad for taxpayers, Perry said, acknowledging that these are questions that are "too uncomfortable for most people to contemplate."

During his time in politics, Perry said, there were advances, such as the focus Harcourt put on settling treaties with BC's Indigenous communities. While it was morally the right thing to do, he said, "Part of the underlying notion was that … the reason to do this is it will improve the lives of people and we won't end up with the devastated communities." The idea was that access to land and more self-determination would help people heal.

But in terms of a wider view on health, it didn't tend to get raised, Perry said. "Who the hell discusses these things within the power centres of government?" The push would tend to come from outside of government, he said. "Real improvements don't come from the top. They come from the bottom." Even as the health critic, Perry found himself supporting issues the health unions were raising criticizing the government that weren't necessarily in the wider public interest, he said. "Like everyone else, I was setting the stage for more money for them that have."

Writing two decades ago, Jonathan Lomas, who taught health policy analysis at McMaster University, and economist André-Pierre Contandriopoulos at the University of Montreal considered who benefited from the status quo. In interactions with patients, given how they are paid, it's clearly in physicians' interest to reinforce the belief that medical care is the best option to help with whatever might be wrong with someone:

In a fee-for-service environment, the physician's income depends on the number of people seeking care, and the quantity of services he or she offers. And if, through processes over which most physicians have little control, the supply of physicians is being increased relative to the population, then on average each person in the population must receive more services, not less, if each physician's workload is not to fall.

And it's not just the doctors who benefit, they wrote. Many people depend on the sickness care industry for their salary. "Behind the physician stands the drug company, and the medical equipment manufacturer, and even the biomedical researcher, all of whom depend for their incomes on expanding the scope of medical intervention," Lomas and Contandriopoulos wrote. "Powerful commercial interests, unconstrained by the professional ethics that may influence the physician's behaviour, place heavy and continuing pressure on physician and patient alike, to find and treat a medical problem, but also to interpret 'health' in as broad terms as possible." There's great incentive to medicalize, and profit from, many conditions that were previously considered within the range of normal human experience. In the words of the authors, "Any perceived inadequacy or unhappiness is a 'health deficit,' which should be treated through medical intervention, since the absence of health is obviously illness. The commodities necessary for such treatment are heavily promoted to physicians and increasingly to patients as well."

The marketing of "cures" extends outside of the medical world, of course. "The calls to jog, to eat better, to stop smoking are everywhere," Lomas and Contandriopoulos wrote. "Such marketing involves, indeed demands, the individualization and medicalization of the target problem. Individual responsibility is emphasized, the victim is blamed, and guilt can be assuaged by purchasing the health club membership or the fat-free meat. Always, however, the message is detached from its social context." Companies will market "cholesterol-free" potato chips or pills to reduce individuals' cholesterol, "but cheerfully leave unaddressed the stress of the workplace hierarchy or the lack of companionship and support for the widowed elderly."

Another part of the problem that Lomas and Contandriopoulos identified was that focusing on the health of a population instead of individuals is relatively abstract and difficult. The factors that contribute to the health of a population are often invisible at the individual level, leading people to misunderstand what really makes them healthy. They wrote:

> For quite understandable reasons, the average person is led to overestimate the effects of medical care on health, and to underestimate the effects of more general social interventions. The latter can be observed at the population level; the former often cannot. But individuals observe their own experience and that of other individuals; they do not see populations.[7]

Besides, environmental and social factors often take time to affect the health of a population. If smoking levels rise, for example, the increased number of cases of lung disease won't be seen for decades. Failure to support families will translate into worse outcomes for their children sometime in the future, not immediately.

There have been, however, some positive signs in Canada in recent years. When Justin Trudeau's Liberal Party formed government in 2015, his mandate letter to Philpott may have ignored the social determinants of health, as mentioned earlier. But the prime minister's mandate letters to other ministers did include further goals aimed at improving health. For example, Trudeau's letter to the minister of Indigenous and northern affairs, Carolyn Bennett, said, "I expect you to re-engage in a renewed nation-to-nation process with Indigenous Peoples to make real progress on the issues most important to First Nations, the Métis Nation, and Inuit communities—issues like housing, employment, health and mental health care, community safety and policing, child welfare, and education." There was to be more funding for First Nations communities, support for child care, and she was to "Make significant new investments in First Nations education to ensure that First Nations children on reserve receive a quality education while respecting the principle of First Nations control of First Nations education." And along with the health minister, Bennett was to "update and expand" the Nutrition North program.[8]

The minister of families, children and social development, Yves Duclos, was to redesign funding for families through the Canada child benefit program, fix the employment insurance system, improve income security for seniors, and lead the development of a poverty reduction strategy for the country. "Our strategy will align with and support existing provincial and municipal poverty reduction strategies," Trudeau's letter for Duclos said. Duclos was also to help make parental leave more flexible and re-establish the federal government's commitment to affordable housing.[9] Infrastructure and Communities Minister Amarjeet Sohi was to work on a ten-year plan to help other levels of government with infrastructure that would include public transit, but also "social infrastructure, including affordable housing, seniors' facilities, early learning and child care, and cultural and recreational infrastructure."[10]

Two years in, there appeared to have been progress on several fronts. Child benefits had been redesigned in a way that gave 90 percent of families more money, and further changes to the program were promised. Consultations on a poverty reduction strategy were underway and an advisory committee remained in the plans. A National Housing Strategy included a commitment of $4 billion over a decade and a goal of reducing chronic homelessness by 50 percent. Canada had officially adopted the United Nations Declaration on the Rights of Indigenous Peoples, which includes recognition of a right to self-determination. There was still a long way to go to see results, and in some areas it could be tough to separate what was real change from what was merely nice words, but the signals were sunny.

At the provincial level, there have been advances as well. In British Columbia, the province at the forefront of the opioid overdose crisis, the agreement between the Green and NDP caucuses that allowed the NDP to form government in the summer of 2017 included plans to reduce the costs of prescription drugs, introduce a poverty-reduction strategy with legislated targets and timelines, create more affordable housing, and adopt "genuine progress" indicators. The new government announced a $100-a-month increase to social assistance rates, and committed to piloting a basic-income program, creating a homelessness action plan and raising the minimum wage to $15 per hour. The agreement also said the government would "increase the emphasis on preventative health initiatives and services."[11]

The provincial health minister, Adrian Dix, has said his goal is to take an approach that reduces inequality. "If we know anything about the social determinants of health, it's that reducing inequality is central to an effort to address both chronic disease and its impacts on British Columbians."[12]

The direction set out in the Green–NDP agreement was promising, but not enough, doctor and public health promoter Trevor Hancock wrote. While there was much to like in the new government's plans to address poverty and housing, he found the agenda on public health fell short. "They still seem to equate health with health care," he said. "The NDP platform makes no mention of wellness, no reference to obesity, tobacco or alcohol—all major causes of disease and premature death—and only a brief commitment to prevention, mainly in the area of mental health." Nor was there any plan to deal with urban sprawl or build healthy communities, he said. The Green Party's belief that "prevention is better than cure" and plan to find a better balance between acute care and prevention was preferable, he wrote.[13]

Other provinces were also taking some positive steps, including moves to adopt higher minimum wages in Ontario and Alberta and to launch a guaranteed income pilot in Ontario. Like the federal government, every province had either produced or begun working on a poverty reduction strategy. And there were also expectations that the 2018 federal budget would take advantage of Canada's unexpectedly strong economy to address poverty and homelessness. Commentators were advocating for a broad approach that addressed income support, education, training, housing and mental health.[14] Perhaps, after fifty years of saying the right words but sliding backwards, there would finally be more progress.

CHAPTER 12

Better

Acting Together for Healthy Generations

In the time that Canada has existed, the gains to public health have been significant. A Canadian born in 1871, the year the first census was taken after Confederation, could have expected to live not long past her or his fortieth birthday. The life expectancy at birth for women was then 43.7 years and for men it was 41.4 years. By 2013, the figures had nearly doubled, adding about forty years to the life expectancies for both women and men. While there's more to life than its length, longer lifespans are a rough measure of improving health. According to Statistics Canada, which published the figures for Canada's 150th birthday, "This notable increase in life expectancy at birth is attributable to several factors, including improved nutrition and sanitation (including access to safe drinking water), advances in medicine and pharmacology (including immunization, improved technologies and knowledge, including maternal health), and improved access to health care and services." A large share of the gains in Canada were made in the early 1900s when children became less likely to die before they turned five years of age. A baby born in 1871 had a one in three chance of reaching sixty-five years of age. Today the figure is nine out of ten. The gains in the first year are particularly large. Compared to a baby born in 1871, one born today is thirty times more likely to reach their first birthday.[1]

Those changes in mortality through the twentieth century were not, however, due to improved medical care. As researchers Clyde Hertzman,

John Frank and Robert Evans wrote, "The dramatic declines in deaths from particular infectious diseases over the nineteenth and early twentieth centuries occurred in the *absence* of any effective medical therapy." They cited data from the Office of Population Censuses and Surveys from the United Kingdom to conclude, "Life expectancy at birth increased in many now 'developed' countries, roughly from forty to sixty years, with little assistance from individual patient treatment or medically delivered prevention aimed at specific diseases." The gains had instead been made thanks to generally improving conditions, they wrote. "Socioeconomic factors, broadly defined, have a major effect not only on the relative health of groups within a population, but on the health of 'the same' population at different points in time."[2]

It is to those social conditions that we must attend if we are truly interested in maximizing the health of the maximum number of people. We have long known that health inequities are a symptom of social inequities and that at each step up the social hierarchy people are healthier. That inequity is at the root of our most visible health crises today, including the opioid overdose emergency and the relative poor health of the country's original inhabitants. While those who are living in poverty have the worst health, it is also true that the middle classes are sicker than the wealthy. Despite that knowledge, it's to the health care system that we tend to turn for solutions. While the system provides much that is essential—and while there are areas like mental health care and addictions treatment where it could do much more—it also soaks up large amounts of money for services that may offer only marginal gains. Frequently it is applying expensive band-aids to conditions that could have been prevented or delayed with a broader social approach—one that starts with reducing economic inequities.

Today, Canadians live longer on average than Americans by a few years, but we are outlived by people in Japan, Spain, France, Italy, Switzerland, Iceland and several other countries.[3] And we are soon to be passed by the South Koreans. By 2030, a girl born in South Korea will have the longest life expectancy in the world at ninety-one years, according to a study published in *The Lancet*.[4] The lead researcher, Majid Ezzati from Imperial College London, was quoted in press reports saying education, nutrition and low levels of obesity, along with investments in universal health care in South Korea would make the difference. "It's basically the opposite of what we're doing in the West, where there's a lot of austerity and inequality."[5] In wealthy countries like Canada, of course, we have options. There's nothing preventing us from choosing to reinvest in social services and taking steps to reduce inequality.

The knowledge that the roots of health lie outside the system that looks after illness, and that public policy matters, has a long history. One of the classic quotes in the field comes from Rudolf Virchow, who besides contributing to medical know-how as a scientist, was prominent in German politics: "Medicine is social science and politics is nothing but medicine on a larger scale."[6] The quote dates from an 1848 essay written around the same time that Hungarian-born Ignaz Semmelweis was in Vienna discovering the difference that hand washing made in controlling the spread of infections in obstetrical clinics.

Systems to provide clean water and safely remove sewage have been used in some places for thousands of years, but the Canadian Public Health Association (CPHA) traces the "true beginnings" of public health to the fourteenth century, when Europeans were trying to limit the spread of plague. "One of the first documented actions was in Venice around 1348, with the appointment of three guardians of public health to detect and exclude ships with passengers infected with that disease," a CPHA report said. Other cities instituted forty-day quarantines on travellers to protect against the spread of infection to local people. A few centuries later, in 1790, Johan Peter Frank connected public health to social justice when he observed that "curative and preventive measures had little impact on populations where people lived in abject poverty and squalor."

There have since been efforts to pasteurize milk, manage the conditions that allow tuberculosis to spread and control the transmission of sexually transmitted diseases. Provision of vitamin C has protected against scurvy and health officials have campaigned against public exposure to lead and other poisonous materials. "Through the 20th century, an expansion of focus from a principally communicable disease perspective to one combining communicable and non-communicable illnesses has broadened public health practice," according to the CPHA.

Despite mistakes made along the way by people acting in the name of public health, "at times clouded by the beliefs of the day," it said, "the goal of these changes and this expansion has always been to foster the health of people and to develop a strong, resilient and just society."[7] Today the dominant thinking in the public health field recognizes the need to work towards adjusting societal structures, particularly for populations at risk, even if that's proven harder for officials to act on. After centuries of success, we appear to have stalled on the cusp of the next great health revolution.

A strong argument for taking the next step is rooted in human rights. As the World Health Organization's constitution puts it, attaining the highest standard of health possible is "one of the fundamental rights of every human being without distinction of race, religion, political belief, economic or social condition."[8] That health is a fundamental right is something we agree with as Canadians, at least officially. As a signatory of the Universal Declaration of Human Rights, proclaimed and adopted by the United Nations General Assembly in 1948, Canada agreed that "Everyone has the right to life, liberty and security of person." We also officially agreed that:

> Everyone has the right to a standard of living adequate for the health and well-being of himself and of his family, including food, clothing, housing and medical care and necessary social services, and the right to security in the event of unemployment, sickness, disability, widowhood, old age or other lack of livelihood in circumstances beyond his control.

And considering how much a person's childhood experiences affect her or his health throughout life, it's worth noting the declaration's confirmation that "Motherhood and childhood are entitled to special care and assistance. All children, whether born in or out of wedlock, shall enjoy the same social protection."[9]

Canada has also ratified the United Nations Convention on the Rights of the Child, which takes the discussion a step further. Signing the convention in 1991 extended Canada's responsibility to provide support for children and their families, the Canadian Public Health Association argued in a position paper. "The Convention recognizes that children are entitled to basic human rights that permit them to survive, develop and thrive, and that governments have a responsibility to provide and protect these rights," the paper said. "It includes the right to a standard of living that is adequate to ensure the child's physical, mental, spiritual, moral and social development." Parents play a crucial role in looking after their children's needs, yes, but governments are responsible to provide programs and services that help parents fulfill their role. "This responsibility should include the provision of adequate childcare of a quality that supports the child's development."[10] It should also be interpreted to include sufficient support for the child's family, since poor children of course live in poor families.

Allowing children to grow up in want, as we have allowed one in five to do in Canada in recent years, is an obvious violation of their human rights. While we sometimes assume there's little to be done about the situation, it would be a mistake to dismiss it as random or an accident. As author and doctor Paul Farmer has written, "Rights violations are, rather, symptoms of deeper pathologies of power and are linked intimately to the social conditions that so often determine who will suffer abuse and who will be shielded from harm."[11] If we are failing children in Canada, and continuing a cycle where many are unlikely to grow into healthy adults, it is only because it serves somebody's interests.

No doubt there are strong forces working against making the changes that would produce a healthier society. When Wei-Ching Chang and Joy Fraser considered the poor success thus far in achieving equity in health, they identified a fundamental problem. "The reason, we suggest, is that we have been reluctant to criticize the culture of competition, which engenders social inequality and health inequity," they wrote in an article for the *International Journal for Equity in Health*. An economic system that relies on the "invisible hand" and pits people against each other in a struggle for either resources or the latest gadget is *set up* to deliver social inequality, and therefore health inequity. To make people healthier, therefore, requires a total reorganization of the economy and adoption of a culture of cooperation, they argued. "Clearly, if our vision includes health equity and health for all, it is logical for us to choose the cooperation over the competition paradigm. Only by creating this paradigm shift will we be edging closer to our cherished vision of health and health equity for all."[12] Acting on the vision would mean a total reordering of the economy, putting cooperation at its centre.

Others have held up hope for making improvements within the economic system we have. As Vancouver doctor Gabor Maté has put it, "It's not necessary to overthrow capitalism to have some better policies. It's not a given that we have to be as stupid as we are."[13]

Certainly, better public policy choices at times seem possible. There is political interest in tackling the interlinked issues of poverty, addiction, homelessness and mental health, but little that could be considered a coordinated response aimed at preventing problems before they develop. For all the good intentions, we often seem to remain stuck in the kind of thinking that got us to where we are today.

I had the opportunity to hear Samantha Nutt speak in late 2016. A family physician and public health specialist, she was founder and executive director of the group War Child Canada. She also knows something about politics, having observed it up close: her husband Eric Hoskins was the health minister in Ontario's Liberal government. In her speech she mentioned the "rising tide of individualism" and the challenge it presented, so later I asked her what she meant. "We make choices often, and we will make even policy choices, based on what's good for the individual as opposed to what's good for society," she said, giving the example of tax cuts. "We have this Reagan-inspired kind of ethos, especially if you're trying to get elected, that taxes are always bad, that taxes are sort of something that's being done to us against our better judgment." But in reality, the money taxes raise is needed and without them we couldn't do any of the things we need to do together. "If we believe in a society that provides for the vulnerable, that supports universal health care, that believes in strengthening our communities and providing those kinds of protections and opportunities, if we believe in an inclusive Canada, then we shouldn't look at tax as an evil, we should look at it as a necessary part of being a good citizen." While we *are* individuals, we are also much more than that. We are family members, neighbours, community members and citizens.

Communicating what it would take to become a healthier society is essential. In Nutt's assessment, people tend to lack a vision for the kind of country they want to live in, making it easy for politicians to pander to our basest instincts. But citizens who share an understanding of how life could be made better for the many can demand action from the politicians who represent them. The politicians, seeing the parade forming, will have little choice but to clamour to get to its head.

The shift starts with individuals understanding that they will themselves be healthier if they live in a society that is healthier overall. As Nutt put it, "Everything for me is really about how we build healthy communities and how we provide the maximum amount of benefit to the largest amount of people." We can become a healthier country, but it requires making that our collective aim and demanding action on it together. The vision laid out decades ago in the Lalonde report, discussed in my first chapter, remains as relevant today as when it was first articulated. While Lalonde's prescription and similar ones that followed were never put into action, over the years the need for them has only grown. Those inclusive ideas, and the commitment to implement them, are needed now more than ever.

Endnotes

EPIGRAPHS

1   Reprinted with permission of the Publisher from *A Healthy Society* by Ryan Meili © Ryan Meili 2018. All rights reserved by the Publisher.

INTRODUCTION

1   Accessed at http://www.who.int/about/mission/en/ on June 15, 2017.

CHAPTER 1

1   Heart and Stroke Foundation of Canada website. Accessed at www.heartandstroke.ca on August 17, 2017.
2   Accessed at www.diabetes.ca on August 17, 2017.
3   Accessed at https://www.ontario.ca/page/healthy-choices on August 17, 2017.
4   Accessed at https://fondationchagnon.org/en/what-we-support/communities/communities-current/quebec-en-forme-healthy-lifestyle.aspx on August 17, 2017.
5   Accessed at https://www.canada.ca/en/health-canada/services/healthy -living.html on August 17, 2017.
6   Timothy Caulfield, *The Cure for Everything* (Toronto: Penguin, 2012), 211.

7   Marc Lalonde, *A New Perspective on the Health of Canadians: A Working Document* (Ottawa: April 1974). Accessed at http://www.phac-aspc.gc.ca /ph-sp/pdf/perspect-eng.pdf.

8   Canadian Institute for Health Information website. Accessed at https:// www.cihi.ca/en/health-spending on August 3, 2017.

9   Trevor Hancock. "Beyond Health Care: From Public Health Policy to Healthy Public Policy." *Canadian Journal of Public Health.* May/June 1985, 9–11.

10 Trevor Hancock, "Why Did Mary Die? Dig Deep to Find Causes," *Times Colonist*, September 6, 2017, A8.

11 Theodore Marmor, Morris Barer and Robert Evans, "The Determinants of a Population's Health: What Can Be Done to Improve a Democratic Nation's Health Status?" *Why Are Some People Healthy and Others Not? The Determinants of Health of Populations*, eds. Robert G. Evans, Morris L. Barer and Theodore R. Marmor (New York: Aldine De Gruyter, 1994), 223.

12 J. Epp, *Achieving Health for All: A Framework for Health Promotion* (Ottawa: Health and Welfare Canada, 1986). Accessed at Health Canada website: https://www.canada.ca/en/health-canada/services/health-care -system/reports-publications/health-care-system/achieving-health -framework-health-promotion.html.

13 National Forum on Health, *Canada Health Action: Building on the Legacy*. Accessed at https://www.canada.ca/en/health-canada/services /health-care-system/reports-publications/health-care-renewal/canada -health-action-building-legacy-volume1.html on August 28, 2017.

14 Andrew Jackson, "Beware the Canadian Austerity Model" (Canadian Centre for Policy Alternatives, June 1, 2010). Accessed at https://www .policyalternatives.ca/publications/monitor/beware-canadian-austerity- model on September 23, 2017.

15 *Healthy People 2000: National Health Promotion and Disease Prevention Objectives* (Boston: Jones and Bartlett Publishers, 1992).

16 Centers for Disease Control and Prevention: National Center for Health Statistics, "Obesity and Overweight." Accessed at https://www.cdc.gov/ nchs/fastats/obesity-overweight.htm on August 3, 2017.

17 Canadian Institute for Health Information, *Trends in Income-Related Health Inequalities in Canada: Summary Report*, November 2015.

Accessed at https://www.cihi.ca/en/summary_report_inequalities_2015_
en.pdf on July 25, 2017.

18   Michael Marmot and Fraser Mustard, "Coronary Heart Disease from a
      Population Perspective," *Why Are Some People Healthy and Others Not?
      The Determinants of Health of Populations*, eds. Robert G. Evans, Morris L.
      Barer and Theodore R. Marmor (New York: Aldine De Gruyter, 1994), 204.

19   Juha Mikkonen and Dennis Raphael, *Social Determinants of Health: The
      Canadian Facts* (Toronto: York University School of Health Policy and
      Management, 2010). Accessed at http://www.thecanadianfacts.org/The
      _Canadian_Facts.pdf.

20   Ibid.

21   Jane Philpott, "30 things I've learned in 30 years as a doctor," Dr. Jane
      Philpott blog, August 24, 2014. Accessed at http://janephilpott.ca
      /30-things-ive-learned-in-30-years-as-a-doctor/ on August 28, 2017.

22   Accessed at http://pm.gc.ca/eng/minister-health-mandate-letter on
      August 10, 2017.

CHAPTER 2

1   Graham Slaughter, "Canadian Doctor Shows Off Her Health Card at
      Bernie Sanders' Medicare Bill Launch," *CTV News*, September 13, 2017.
      Accessed at http://www.ctvnews.ca/canada/canadian-doctor-shows-off
      -her-health-card-at-bernie-sanders-medicare-bill-launch-1.3588306 on
      September 17, 2017.

2   Eric C. Schneider et al., *Mirror, Mirror 2017: International Comparison
      Reflects Flaws and Opportunities for Better U.S. Health Care*
      (The Commonwealth Fund, July 2017). Accessed at http://www
      .commonwealthfund.org/~/media/files/publications/fund-report/2017/jul
      /schneider_mirror_mirror_2017.pdf on August 2, 2017.

3   Matthew Stanbrook, "Why the Federal Government Must Lead in Health
      Care," *Canadian Medical Association Journal*, August 17, 2015.

4   Canadian Health Coalition, "Everyone Needs to Give During Today's
      Health Accord Talks." Received December 19, 2016, by email.

5   Canadian Health Coalition, "Canadian Health Advocates to Premiers:
      Stand up for Public Health Care." Received July 19, 2017, by email.

6   Accessed at http://www.healthcoalition.ca/about-us/team/ on July 21, 2017.

7   Gloria Galloway, "NDP Vows to Make Health Top Priority," *The Globe and Mail*, September 8, 2016.

CHAPTER 3

1   Wendy Levinson, "Over One Million Canadians Get Unneeded Tests," *The Province*, April 30, 2017, A26.

2   George Carson and Wendy Levinson, "Too Many Medical Procedures on Women Aren't Necessary," *Toronto Star*, June 25, 2017. Accessed at https://www.thestar.com/opinion/commentary/2017/06/25/too-many-medical-procedures-on-women-arent-necessary.html on June 26, 2017.

3   "WHO Statement on Caesarean Section Rates." Accessed at http://www.who.int/reproductivehealth/publications/maternal_perinatal_health/cs-statement/en/ on November 18, 2017.

4   George Carson and Wendy Levinson, "Too Many Medical Procedures on Women Aren't Necessary."

5   Kelly Grant, "Study Highlights Unneeded Medical Care," *The Globe and Mail*, April 7, 2017, A10.

6   Alan Cassels, *Seeking Sickness: Medical Screening and the Misguided Hunt for Disease* (Vancouver, BC: Greystone Books, 2012).

7   Accessed at http://www.oncologynurseadvisor.com/prostate-cancer/prostate-specific-antigen-psa-test-fact-sheet/article/471199/2/ on September 17, 2017.

8   Accessed at http://www.cancer.ca/en/cancer-information/diagnosis-and-treatment/tests-and-procedures/prostate-specific-antigen-psa/ on November 19, 2017.

9   Wendy Levinson, "Over One Million Canadians Get Unneeded Tests."

10 Michelle McQuigge, "Many Tests on Patients a Waste of Time: Study," *Times Colonist*, April 7, 2017, C1.

11 Wendy Levinson, "Over One Million Canadians Get Unneeded Tests."

12 Donald Berwick and Andrew Hackbarth, "Eliminating Waste in US Health Care," *Journal of the American Medical Association*, 2012, 307(14):1513–1516. doi:10.1001/jama.2012.362.

13 Kelly Grant, "Study Highlights Unneeded Medical Care."

14 The Dartmouth Atlas of Health Care, "Reflections on Variations." Accessed at http://www.dartmouthatlas.org/keyissues/issue .aspx?con=1338 on September 3, 2017.

15 Trevor Hancock, "The Secret of Medicine Is Masterly Inactivity," *Times Colonist*, November 16, 2016, A8.

16 Norman J. Temple and Joy Fraser. "Modern Western Medicine: Lots of Bucks—Where's the Bang?" *Exce$$ive Medical $pending*, 106.

17 Theodore Marmor, Morris Barer and Robert Evans. "The Determinants of a Population's Health: What Can Be Done to Improve a Democratic Nation's Health Status?" *Why Are Some People Healthy and Others Not? The Determinants of Health of Populations.* Eds. Robert G. Evans, Morris L. Barer and Theodore R. Marmor (New York: Aldine De Gruyter, 1994), 217.

18 Norman J. Temple and Andrew Thompson, *Exce$$ive Medical $pending: Facing the Challenge* (Oxford: Radcliffe Publishing, 2007).

19 Auditor General of British Columbia, *Health Funding Explained 2*, March 2017. Accessed at http://www.bcauditor.com/pubs on March 14, 2017.

20 Daniel J. Dutton, Pierre-Gerlier Forest, Ronald D. Kneebone and Jennifer D. Zwicker. "Effect of Provincial Spending on Social Services and Health Care on Health Outcomes in Canada: An Observational Longitudinal Study." *Canadian Medical Association Journal*, January 22, 2018.

21 Norman J. Temple and Andrew Thompson, *Exce$$ive Medical $pending*.

22 Atul Gawande, "Tell Me Where it Hurts," *New Yorker*, January 23, 2017: 36–45.

23 Norman J. Temple and Andrew Thompson, *Exce$$ive Medical $pending*.

24 Insights West, "Nurses, Doctors and Scientists Are Canada's Most Respected Professionals." Received June 15, 2017, by email.

25 Audrey Balay-Karperien, Norman Temple and Joel Lexchin, "The Marketing of Drugs: How Drug Companies Manipulate the Prescribing Habits of Doctors," *Exce$$ive Medical $pending*.

26 Accessed at http://www.parl.gc.ca/HousePublications/Publication.aspx ?Language=e&Mode=1&Parl=42&Ses=1&DocId=8651955 on December 30, 2016.

27 Therapeutics Initiative, "Is Cyclobenzaprine Useful for Pain?" July 24, 2017. Accessed at https://www.ti.ubc.ca/2017/07/24/105-cyclobenzaprine/ on September 22, 2017.

28 Matthew Herper, "The World's Most Expensive Drugs," *Forbes*, February 22, 2010. Accessed at https://www.forbes.com/2010/02/19/expensive -drugs-cost-business-healthcare-rare-diseases.html on September 21, 2017.

29 Katie DeRosa, "$250,000-a-Year Drug Focus of Insurance Fight," *Times Colonist*, September 22, 2017, A3.

30 Eike-Henner Kluge, "Health Ministry Has to Make Hard Choices," *Times Colonist*, October 1, 2017, A11.

31 Norman J. Temple and Joy Fraser. "Modern Western Medicine: Lots of Bucks—Where's the Bang?" *Exce$$ive Medical $pending*.

32 Norman J. Temple, "Disease Prevention: The Neglected Alternative," *Exce$$ive Medical $pending*.

33 Jeffrey Simpson, *Chronic Condition: Why Canada's Health-Care System Needs to Be Dragged into the 21st Century* (Toronto: Allen Lane, 2012).

34 Accessed at http://www.budget.gc.ca/2017/docs/plan/anx-01-en .html#Toc477707537 on July 30, 2017.

35 André Picard, *Matters of Life and Death* (Madeira Park, BC: Douglas & McIntyre, 2017).

36 Reprinted with permission of the Publisher from *A Healthy Society* by Ryan Meili © Ryan Meili 2018. All rights reserved by the Publisher.

37 Ryan Meili, *A Healthy Society: How a Focus on Health Can Revive Canadian Democracy* (Saskatoon, SK: Purich Publishing Ltd., 2012).

38 Public Health Agency of Canada, *The Direct Economic Burden of Socio-Economic Health Inequalities in Canada* (Ottawa, 2016).

39 Iglika Ivanova, *The Cost of Poverty in BC* (Canadian Centre for Policy Alternatives, BC Office, July 2011). Accessed at https://www .policyalternatives.ca/sites/default/files/uploads/publications/BC %20Office/2011/07/CCPA_BC_cost_of_poverty_full_report.pdf on August 25, 2017.

CHAPTER 4

1 Accessed at http://www.torontohealthprofiles.ca/a_documents/TM_ allCateg_maps/TM_maps_PM/1_PM_0-74_MF_N_2006-2008_Rate _PWQ.pdf on September 17, 2017.

2   Sandro Galea, "Health in New York and Chicago by Subway and L-Stops: A Pictorial Essay" (Boston University School of Public Health, May 17, 2015). Accessed at https://www.bu.edu/sph/2015/05/17/health-in-new -york-and-chicago-by-subway-and-l-stops-a-pictorial-essay/ on July 10, 2017.

3   Robert Wood Johnson Foundation, "City Maps," September 11, 2015. Accessed at http://www.rwjf.org/en/library/articles-and-news/2015/09/ city-maps.html on July 10, 2017.

4   Olivia Egen et al., "Health and Social Conditions of the Poorest Versus Wealthiest Counties in the United States," *American Journal of Public Health*, December 7, 2016. Accessed at http://ajph.aphapublications.org/ doi/abs/10.2105/AJPH.2016.303515 on July 26, 2017.

5   Ronnie Cohen, "Richest Americans Live Seven to 10 Years Longer than Poorest," Reuters Health, December 5, 2016. Accessed at http://www .reuters.com/article/us-health-lifeexpectancy-wealth-idUSKBN13U200 on July 15, 2017.

6   Amartya Sen, "Foreword," *Pathologies of Power: Health, Human Rights, and the New War on the Poor* (Berkeley, CA: University of California Press, 2003).

7   Statistics Canada, "Archived—Life Expectancy at Birth, by Sex, by Province." Accessed at http://www.statcan.gc.ca/tables-tableaux/sum -som/l01/cst01/health26-eng.htm on July 20, 2017.

8   Statistics Canada, "Canadian Community Health Survey, 2015," March 22, 2017. Accessed at http://www.statcan.gc.ca/daily-quotidien/170322/ dq170322a-eng.htm on March 22, 2017.

9   University of British Columbia, My Health My Community. Accessed at https://www.myhealthmycommunity.org/Results/NeighbourhoodProfiles .aspx on July 10, 2017.

10   Provincial Health Services Authority, *Priority Health Equity Indicators for British Columbia: Selected Indicators Report* (Vancouver, BC: Provincial Health Services Authority, Population and Public Health Program, 2016). Accessed at http://www.phsa.ca/population-public-health-site/ Documents/Priority%20health%20equity%20indicators%20for%20BC _selected%20indicators%20report_2016.pdf on July 20, 2017.

11   Tom Blackwell and Monika Warzecha, "A Country Divided," *Vancouver Sun*, May 8, 2017, N2.

12   Direct Testimony on behalf of BCOAPO, BCUC Project No. 3698781. Accessed at http://www.bcuc.com/Documents/Proceedings/2016/DOC _46279_C2-12_BCOAPO-Intervener-Evidence.pdf on May 25, 2016.

13   Randy Shore, "Cost a Factor in Filling Drug Prescriptions," *Vancouver Sun*, February 2, 2017, A7.

14   David J. T. Campbell et al., "Self-Reported Financial Barriers to Care among Patients with Cardiovascular-Related Chronic Conditions," Statistics Canada. Accessed at http://www.statcan.gc.ca/pub/82-003-x /2014005/article/14005-eng.htm on September 17, 2017.

15   CBC News, "Treating Poverty Works Like Medicine, Doctors Say: Financial Support Can Pay Off with Better Health," May 26, 2013. Accessed at http://www.cbc.ca/news/health/treating-poverty-works-like -medicine-doctors-say-1.1365662 on July 28, 2017.

16   Timothy Caulfield, *The Cure for Everything*, 76.

17   Juha Mikkonen and Dennis Raphael, *Social Determinants of Health*.

18   Food Banks Canada, Hunger Count 2016 (2016).

19   © Richard and Kate Pickett, 2009, *The Spirit Level: Why Equality is Better for Everyone*, Bloomsbury Press, an imprint of Bloomsbury Publishing Inc.

20   Statistics Canada, "Health Fact Sheets: Fruit and Vegetable Consumption, 2015," March 22, 2017. Accessed at http://www.statcan.gc.ca/pub/82-625-x/2017001/article/14764-eng.htm on September 17, 2017.

21   George Orwell, *The Road to Wigan Pier* (Harmondsworth, England: Penguin Books, 1975). (Copyright 1937.)

22   Marc Renaud, "The Future: Hygeia versus Panakeia?" *Why are Some People Healthy and Others Not? The Determinants of Health of Populations*, eds. Robert G. Evans, Morris L. Barer and Theodore R. Marmor (New York: Aldine De Gruyter, 1994), 318.

23   Statistics Canada, "Canadian Community Health Survey," 2016, September 27, 2017. Accessed at http://www.statcan.gc.ca/daily -quotidien/170927/dq170927a-eng.htm on September 27, 2017.

24   World Health Organization, "Social Determinants of Health." Accessed at http://www.who.int/social_determinants/thecommission/interview _marmot/en/ on June 15, 2017.

25   Michael Tjepkema, Russell Wilkins and Andrea Long, *Cause-Specific Mortality by Income Adequacy in Canada: A 16-Year Follow-Up Study*,

Statistics Canada. Accessed at http://www.statcan.gc.ca/pub/82-003-x /2013007/article/11852-eng.htm on August 14, 2017.

26 Dennis Raphael and Toba Bryant, "Income Inequality Is Killing Thousands of Canadians Every Year," *Toronto Star*, November 23, 2014. Accessed at https://www.thestar.com/opinion/commentary/2014/11/23/ income_inequality_is_killing_thousands_of_canadians_every_year.html on August 16, 2017.

CHAPTER 5

1 M. Chartier et al., *The Mental Health of Manitoba's Children* (Winnipeg, MB: Manitoba Centre for Health Policy, Fall 2016).

2 David Heft, "Mental Health-Care Services Quietly Eroding," *Times Colonist*, February 7, 2017, A11.

3 Accessed at http://www.cbc.ca/radio/thecurrent/the-current-for -february-2-2017-1.3962070/you-can-t-look-away-from-a-smell -a-reporter-s-struggle-with-ptsd-1.3962105 on June 23, 2017.

4 Statistics Canada, "Families, Households and Marital Status: Key Results from the 2016 Census," August 2, 2017. Accessed at http://www.statcan. gc.ca/daily-quotidien/170802/dq170802a-eng.htm on August 2, 2017.

5 Dhruv Khullar, "Social Isolation Is a Growing Epidemic, One That's Increasingly Recognized as Having Dire Physical, Mental and Emotional Consequences," *New York Times*, December 22, 2016. Accessed at https:// www.nytimes.com/2016/12/22/upshot/how-social-isolation-is-killing-us. html on July 3, 2017.

6 Gloria Levi and Laura Kadawaki, *Our Future: Seniors, Socialization, and Health* (Vancouver, BC: Columbia Institute, April 2016). Accessed at http://www.civicgovernance.ca/wordpress/wp-content/uploads/2016/04/ Columbia_Seniors_April_2016_web.pdf on June 20, 2017.

7 Statistics Canada, "Canadian Tobacco Alcohol and Drugs (CTADS): 2013 Summary." Accessed at http://healthycanadians.gc.ca/science-research -sciences-recherches/data-donnees/ctads-ectad/summary-sommaire -2013-eng.php on June 23, 2017.

8 Statistics Canada, "Heavy Drinking, 2013." Accessed at http://www.statcan. gc.ca/pub/82-625-x/2014001/article/14019-eng.htm on June 23, 2017.

9   Accessed at https://www.mapleridge.ca/962/Nicole-Read on September 22, 2017.

10   Robert Duffy, Gaetan Royer and Charley Beresford, *Who's Picking Up the Tab? Federal and Provincial Downloading onto Local Governments* (Vancouver: Columbia Institute Centre for Civic Governance, September 2014).

11   Sarah Petrescu, "B.C. Spent $3 Million on Tent City, Papers Show," *Times Colonist*, Thursday, August 3, 2017, A1.

12   Metro Vancouver, *Addressing Homelessness in Metro Vancouver*, February 2017. Accessed at http://www.metrovancouver.org/services/regional -planning/homelessness/homelessness-taskforce/plan/Documents/ HomelessnessStrategy2017.pdf on August 15, 2017.

13   The Canadian Press, "Homelessness in Canada: Key Statistics," *CTV News*, March 16, 2016. Accessed at http://www.ctvnews.ca/canada/ homelessness-in-canada-key-statistics-1.2819986 on August 18, 2017.

14   Social Solutions, "2016's Shocking Homelessness Statistics." Accessed at http://www.socialsolutions.com/blog/2016-homelessness-statistics/ on August 18, 2017.

15   Alastair Gee, Liz Barney and Julia O'Malley, "How America Counts Its Homeless—and Why So Many Are Overlooked," *The Guardian*, February 16, 2017. Accessed at https://www.theguardian.com/us-news/2017/feb/16/ homeless-count-population-america-shelters-people on August 18, 2017.

16   Metro Vancouver, "Addressing Homelessness in Metro Vancouver."

17   Paula Goering et al., *National At Home/Chez Soi Final Report* (Calgary, AB: Mental Health Commission of Canada, 2014). Accessed at http:// www.mentalhealthcommission.ca on September 16, 2017.

18   André Picard, *Matters of Life and Death.*

19   Travis Lupick, "B.C. Manifesto for Better Mental Health Calls for Province to Prioritize Prevention and Support in the Community" *Georgia Straight*, October 11, 2016. Accessed at http://www.straight .com/news/804541/bc-manifesto-better-mental-health-calls-province -prioritize-prevention-and-support on January 10, 2017.

20   Statistics Canada, *Canadian Community Health Survey, 2015.*

CHAPTER 6

1   Jackie Wong, "In Throes of Overdose Crisis, a Community Unites to Fight Back," *The Tyee*, January 1, 2017. Accessed at https://thetyee.ca/ News/2017/01/25/Fighting-Back-Overdose-Crisis/ on July 3, 2017.

2   Ministry of Public Safety and Solicitor General and BC Coroners Service, "June Illicit Drug-Death Numbers." Received August 4, 2017, by email.

3   Meghan Potkins, "Alberta Opioid Crisis 'Completely Out of Hand'," *National Post*, September 5, 2017, A3.

4   Nick Boisvert, "Overdose Calls Jump 28% but Toronto Police Still Aren't Carrying Naloxone Kits," *CBC News*, November 16, 2017. Accessed at http://www.cbc.ca/news/canada/toronto/toronto-police-overdoses-1 .4403603 on November 24, 2017.

5   Dwight Chapin, "How to Treat Chronic Pain without Turning to Opioids."

6   Linda So, "Ohio County Claims Top Spot in America's Opioid Death Spiral," *Reuters*, June 21, 2017. Accessed at https://www.reuters.com/ article/us-usa-opioids-ohio/ohio-county-claims-top-spot-in-americas -opioid-death-spiral-idUSKBN19C2WA on September 16, 2017.

7   BC Coroners Service, Public Safety and Solicitor General, "Statement: International Overdose Awareness Day." Received August 31, 2017, by email.

8   Tina Lovgreen, "Fears of Accidental Exposure to Fentanyl Hamper Efforts of Conservation Groups," *CBC News*, June 13, 2017. Accessed at http:// www.cbc.ca/news/canada/british-columbia/fentanyl-hamper-efforts -conversation-groups-1.4157554 on June 15, 2017.

9   Anthonie den Boef, "Addicts Should Get One Chance," *Vancouver Sun*, January 4, 2017, A9.

10 Tieleman, Bill. "Drug Overdoses Kill Four a Day in BC, and Inaction and Apathy Are to Blame," *The Tyee*, July 11, 2017.

11 Leslie McBain, "My Son's Death Offers Lessons for Ending the Opioid Epidemic," *The Globe and Mail*, September 1, 2017, S1.

12 Kristy Kirkup, "B.C. Officials Eye Portugal's Drug Policy," *The Globe and Mail*, August 10, 2017, S2.

13 Mike Hager, "Ottawa Rejects Expert Calls to Decriminalize Illegal Opioids," *The Globe and Mail*, August 28, 2017, S1.

14   Jackie Wong, "An Urgent Call on Overdose Crisis: Prescribe Drugs, End Prohibition," *The Tyee*, January 26, 2017. Accessed at https://thetyee.ca/News/2017/01/26/Prescribe-Drugs-End-Prohibition/ on June 25, 2017.

15   Dwight Chapin, "How to Treat Chronic Pain without Turning to Opioids."

16   Tom Blackwell, "'This Is A Lesson': One Paragraph May Have Triggered Opioid Crisis," *National Post*, June 1, 2017, A1.

17   Evan Wood, "Opioid Crisis Calls for Smarter Prescribing," *The Globe and Mail*, July 27, 2017, S2.

18   Diane Peters, "Charismatic Guru Popularized Ancient Ideas," *The Globe and Mail*, July 29, 2017, S16.

19   Kenneth Tupper, "How to Stem Overdose Cases," *Vancouver Sun*, August 12, 2017, B2.

20   Kate Smolina and Kim Rutherford, "Alternatives to Opioids Needed for Chronic Pain Relief," *The Province*, January 30, 2017, A15.

21   Wanyee Li, "Mental Health and Drug Addiction included in Vancouver Police's Top Priorities," *Metro News*. Accessed at metronews.ca on January 24, 2017.

22   Ministry of Public Safety and Solicitor General BC Coroners Service, "Inquest Recommendations Concerning Illicit Drug Death." Received January 25, 2017, by email.

23   Jane Philpott, "Getting to the Root of Canada's Opioid Crisis," *The Globe and Mail*, January 16, 2017, S2.

24   Travis Lupick, "Vancouver Prescription Heroin Users Wage Court Battle with the Feds," *Georgia Straight*, March 19, 2014. Accessed at http://www.straight.com/news/609391/vancouver-prescription-heroin-users-wage-court-battle-feds on July 20, 2017.

25   Jane Philpott, "Getting to the Root of Canada's Opioid Crisis."

26   Peter O'Neil, "Mayors Link Drug Crisis, Housing Need," *Vancouver Sun*, January 21, 2017, A4.

27   Lawrie McFarlane, "'Deaths from Despair' Demand Answers," *Times Colonist*, March 31, 2017, A11.

28   Douglas Todd, "Fentanyl: A Men's Health Crisis," *Vancouver Sun*, March 20, 2017.

29   Andre C. Piver, "Mental-Health Workers Must Be Allowed to Care, Provide Hope," *Vancouver Sun*, March 25, 2017, B4.

30 Jackie Wong, "The Overdose Crisis: We Know How to Save Lives, Doctors Say," *The Tyee*, January 27, 2017. Accessed at https://thetyee.ca/News/2017/01/27/BC-Overdose-Crisis/ on June 25, 2017.

31 Pamela Fayerman, "Judy Darcy: 'I Will Pour My Heart and Soul' into Mental Health/Addictions File," *Vancouver Sun*, July 27, 2017. Accessed at http://vancouversun.com/news/local-news/judy-darcy-i-will-pour-my-heart-and-soul-into-mental-healthaddictions-file on July 27, 2017.

32 Judy Darcy, "Transforming Mental Health and Addictions Care in B.C.," Ministry of Mental Health and Addictions. Received August 16, 2017, by email.

33 Diane McIntosh, "Fentanyl Scourge Tied to Mental Health Crisis," *The Province*, July 2, 2017, A21.

34 Staff, "Path of the Shaman Doc Goes Deep with B.C. Ayahuasca Healer," *Metro News*, Accessed at metronews.ca on May 29, 2017.

35 Isolde Verbrugge, "Consumption Sites Not About Wellness," *Times Colonist*, August 20, 2017, A11.

36 Bruce Alexander, "Addiction: The View from Rat Park (2010)." Accessed at http://www.brucekalexander.com/articles-speeches/rat-park/148-addiction-the-view-from-rat-park on August 30, 2017.

CHAPTER 7

1 Jen St. Denis, "Overdose Crisis Affecting Vancouver's Indigenous at Stunningly High Rate: Chief Medical Officer," *Metro News*. Accessed at metronews.ca on July 26, 2017.

2 Nick Eagland, "First Nations People Three Times More Likely to Die from Overdose, Stats Show," *Vancouver Sun*, August 4, 2017, A8.

3 Andrea Woo, "Overdose Rate Higher among First Nations," *The Globe and Mail*, Friday, August 4, 2017, A4.

4 Katie Hyslop, "First Nations Still Vastly Overrepresented in BC Overdose Deaths," *The Tyee*, August 3, 2017. Accessed at https://thetyee.ca/News/2017/08/03/First-Nations-Overrepresented-BC-Overdose-Deaths/ on August 3, 2017.

5 Jennifer Graham, "Chief Perry Bellegarde Open AFN Meeting with Plea to End Racism, Violence," *The Canadian Press*, July 25, 2017. Accessed

at http://www.ctvnews.ca/canada/chief-perry-bellegarde-opens-afn -meeting-with-plea-to-end-racism-violence-1.3518165 on July 26, 2017.

6 Statistics Canada, "Victimization of Aboriginal people in Canada, 2014," June 28, 2016.

7 Representative for Children and Youth, *Too Many Victims: Sexualized Violence in the Lives of Children and Youth in Care* (Victoria, BC: October 2016).

8 Manon Lamontagne, *Violence Against Aboriginal Women: Scan and Report* (Canadian Women's Foundation, October 31, 2011).

9 Bev Lambert, "In Resolving Addiction, Address the Root Causes," *Times Colonist*, August 4, 2017, A13.

10 Metro Vancouver, *Final Aboriginal Homelessness Report of 2017: Homeless Count in Metro Vancouver Released.* Received September 25, 2017, by email.

11 British Columbia Coroners Service and First Nations Health Authority Death Review Panel, *A Review of First Nation Youth and Young Adult Injury Deaths: 2010–2015* (British Columbia Coroners Service and First Nations Health Authority, November 2017).

12 Statistics Canada, *Canadian Community Health Survey.*

13 Tom Blackwell and Monika Warzecha, "A Country Divided."

14 CBC News, "Canada 'Falls Short' in Treating First Nations Patients, Says Country's 1st Female Indigenous Surgeon," December 13, 2016. Accessed at http://www.cbc.ca/news/health/dr-nadine-caron-indigenous-surgeon -health-1.3887752 on September 22, 2017.

15 Statistics Canada, Study: *Food Insecurity among Inuit Living in Inuit Nunangat*, 2012. Accessed at http://www.statcan.gc.ca/daily-quotidien /170201/dq170201a-eng.htm on August 3, 2017.

16 Ian Mosby and Tracey Galloway, "'Hunger Was Never Absent': How Residential School Diets Shaped Current Patterns of Diabetes among Indigenous Peoples in Canada," *Canadian Medical Association Journal*, August 14, 2017, vol. 189 no. 32 doi:10.1503/cmaj.170448.

17 Accessed at https://foodsecurecanada.org/resources-news/news-media /cost-food-national-food-policy-should-focus-health-and-sustainability on November 25, 2017.

18 Leanna Garfield, "Food Prices Are Insanely High in Rural Canada, where Ketchup Costs $14 and Sunny D Costs $29," *Business Insider*, September

21, 2017. Accessed at http://www.businessinsider.com/food-prices-high
-northern-canada-2017-9/#the-feeding-my-family-facebook-group-hopes
-to-connect-sub-arctic-residents-who-struggle-with-food-insecurity
-from-northern-labrador-in-the-east-to-northern-alaska-in-the-west-1 on
November 25, 2017.

19 Accessed at http://decisions.chrt-tcdp.gc.ca/chrt-tcdp/decisions/en/item
/127700/index.do?r=AAAAAQAKVDEzNDAvNzAwOAE on August
18, 2017.

20 David Ball, "Scared and Spied On Under Harper, Why Child Advocate
Didn't Give Up," *The Tyee*, January 29, 2016. Accessed at www.thetyee.ca
on July 12, 2017.

21 Cindy Blackstock and Sébastien Grammond, "Reforming Child Welfare
First Step Toward Reconciliation: Opinion," *Toronto Star*, August 1, 2017.
Accessed at https://www.thestar.com/opinion/commentary/2017/08/01
/reforming-child-welfare-first-step-toward-reconciliation-opinion.html
on July 12, 2017.

22 Tracy Sherlock, "Cindy Blackstock Says Trudeau Government's 'Making
Excuses' for Neglecting Indigenous Children," *National Observer*, July 31,
2017. Accessed at http://www.nationalobserver.com/2017/07/31/news/
cindy-blackstock-says-trudeau-governments-making-excuses-neglecting
-indigenous on August 3, 2017.

23 Gloria Galloway, "Ottawa Still Failing to Provide Health Care on
Reserves: Report," *The Globe and Mail*, January 25, 2017, A5.

24 Ibid.

25 Jane Philpott, "CMA Speech," Health Canada, August 21, 2017. Accessed
at https://www.canada.ca/en/health-canada/news/2017/08/cma_speech
_-_janephilpott-august212017.html on August 22, 2017.

26 Provincial Health Officer of BC and the First Nations Health Authority,
First Nations Health and Well-Being Interim Update, November 12, 2015.
Accessed at http://www2.gov.bc.ca/assets/gov/health/about-bc-s-health
-care-system/office-of-the-provincial-health-officer/reports-publications
/special-reports/first-nations-health-and-well-being-interim-update-nov
-2015.pdf on July 17, 2017.

27 CBC Radio, *Early Edition*, January 4, 2017. (Interview with Rick Cluff.)

28 Alan Katz, Jennifer Enns and Kathi Avery Kinew, "Canada Needs a
    Holistic First Nations Health Strategy," *Canadian Medical Association
    Journal*, August 8, 2017, 189:E1006-7. doi:10.1503/cmaj.170261.
29 Ibid.

CHAPTER 8

1   Metro Vancouver, "Continued Air Quality Advisory." Received August 1,
    2017, by email.
2   Accessed at weather.gc.ca/airquality/pages/bcaq-010_e.html on August
    3, 2017.
3   Justin McElroy, "Kamloops Experiencing Worst Air Quality in Its
    Recorded History," *CBC News*, August 3, 2017. Accessed at www.cbc.ca
    /news/canada/british-columbia/kamloops-air-quality-1.4234720 on
    August 3, 2017.
4   Staff, "Hospital Visits Spike in B.C. as Smoky Air from Wildfires Lingers,"
    Times Colonist, August 6, 2017, A5.
5   Medical Society Consortium on Climate and Health, *Medical Alert!
    Climate Change Is Harming Our Health*, 2017. Accessed at https://
    medsocietiesforclimatehealth.org/wp-content/uploads/2017/03/medical
    _alert.pdf on August 10, 2017.
6   Accessed at http://www.nrcan.gc.ca/forests/fire-insects-disturbances/
    fire/13155 on August 10, 2017.
7   Medical Society Consortium on Climate and Health, *Medical Alert!*
8   Camilo Mora et al., "Global Risk of Deadly Heat," *Nature Climate Change*,
    June 19, 2017, 7, 501–506. Accessed at https://www.nature.com/nclimate/
    journal/v7/n7/full/nclimate3322.html on August 11, 2017.
9   Ivan Semeniuk, "Scientists Calculate Rising Risk of Lethal Heat Waves,"
    The Globe and Mail, June 20, 2017, A4.
10 Warren Bell and Amy Lubik, "Opinion: B.C.'s Climate Plan Is a Public
    Health Failure," *Vancouver Sun*, September 5, 2016.
11 Marco Springmann et al., "Global and Regional Health Effects of Future
    Food Production under Climate Change: A Modelling Study," *The Lancet*,
    volume 387, issue 10031, 1937–1946. Acccessed at http://www.thelancet

.com/journals/lancet/article/PIIS0140-6736(15)01156-3/abstract on September 24, 2017.

12   Kate Kelland, "Sperm Count Falling Sharply in Developed World, Researchers Say," *Reuters*, July 25, 2017. Accessed at http://www.reuters .com/article/us-health-sperm-idUSKBN1AA28K on August 2, 2017.

13   Canadian Press, "Air Pollution Results in 7,700 Premature Deaths in Canada Each Year, Report Says," *CBC News*, June 1, 2017. Accessed at http://www.cbc.ca/news/health/air-pollution-results-in-7-700-premature -deaths-in-canada-each-year-report-says-1.4140794 on August 24, 2017.

14   World Health Organization, "7 million premature deaths annually linked to air pollution," March 25, 2014. Accessed at http://www.who.int/ mediacentre/news/releases/2014/air-pollution/en/ on August 11, 2017.

15   Hannah Devlin, "Living Near Heavy Traffic Increases Risk of Dementia, Say Scientists," *The Guardian*, January 5, 2017. Accessed at https://www .theguardian.com/society/2017/jan/04/living-near-heavy-traffic-increases -dementia-risk-say-scientists on August 11, 2017.

16   Sarah Knapton, "Car Engine Particles Linked to Alzheimer's," *National Post*, September 6, 2016, A2.

17   Yale School of Public Health, "Fracking Linked to Cancer-Causing Chemicals, New YSPH Study Finds." Accessed at publichealth.yale.edu/ news/article.aspx?id=13714 on October 25, 2016.

18   Canadian Association of Physicians for the Environment, "CAPE Position Statement on Fracking," June 2014. Accessed at https://cape.ca/ wp-content/uploads/2014/06/Fracking-CAPE-Position-Statement-June -2014.pdf on August 31, 2017.

19   Martin Mittelstaedt, "Pollution Debate Born of Chemical Valley's Girl-Baby Boom," *The Globe and Mail*, November 15, 2005. Accessed at https://www.theglobeandmail.com/technology/science/pollution-debate -born-of-chemical-valleys-girl-baby-boom/article18253243/ on December 5, 2017.

20   Benjamin Shingler, "Sarnia Area First Nation Facing Health Problems from Exposure to Pollutants," *Toronto Star* (The Canadian Press), November 24, 2013. Accessed at https://www.thestar.com/news/canada /2013/11/24/sarnia_area_first_nation_facing_health_problems_from _exposure_to_pollutants.html on September 24, 2017.

21   Jonny Wakefield, "'What's in That Fish?' Scientists Set to Launch Major Study of Mercury in Williston Lake," *Dawson Creek Mirror*, May 27, 2016. Accessed at http://www.dawsoncreekmirror.ca/regional-news/site-c/what-s-in-that-fish-scientists-set-to-launch-major-study-of-mercury-in-williston-lake-1.2265230 on September 2, 2017.

22   David Suzuki Foundation and Council of Canadians, *Glass Half Empty? Year 1 Progress Toward Resolving Drinking Water Advisories in Nine First Nations in Ontario*, February 2017.

23   Amy Minsky, "First Nations 'Living in Third World Conditions' as Communities Endure Water Advisories," *Global News*, February 9, 2017. Accessed at http://globalnews.ca/news/3238948/first-nations-drinking-water-crisis-liberals-promise/ on September 2, 2017.

24   Canadian Population Health Initiative, *Summary Report Urban Physical Environments and Health Inequalities*, March 2011. Accessed at https://www.cihi.ca/en/cphi_upe_summary_rep_en.pdf on September 3, 2017.

25   Devra Davis, *The Secret History of the War on Cancer* (New York: Basic Books, 2007).

26   Quoted in Medical Society Consortium on Climate and Health report.

27   World Health Organization, "7 Million Premature Deaths Annually Linked to Air Pollution."

28   Canadian Public Health Association, *Global Change and Public Health: Addressing the Ecological Determinants of Health*, May 2015. Accessed at https://www.cpha.ca/sites/default/files/assets/policy/edh-discussion_e.pdf on August 1, 2017.

CHAPTER 9

1   Doug Kelly, "The Hidden Complexities in Substance Addiction," *The Globe and Mail*, August 25, 2017, S2.

2   Danielle Martin, *Better Now: Six Big Ideas to Improve Health Care for All Canadians* (Canada: Allen Lane, 2017), 191.

3   World Health Organization, "Constitution of WHO: Principles." Accessed at http://www.who.int/about/mission/en/ on July 17, 2017.

4   Lori G. Irwin, Arjumand Siddiqi and Clyde Hertzman, "Early Child Development: A Powerful Equalizer," World Health Organization's

Commission on the Social Determinants of Health, 2007. Accessed at http://www.who.int/social_determinants/resources/ecd_kn_report _07_2007.pdf

5   Robert Evans, Matthew Hodge and Barry Pless, "If Not Genetics, Then What? Biological Pathways and Population Health," *Why are Some People Healthy and Others Not? The Determinants of Health of Populations*, eds. Robert G. Evans, Morris L. Barer and Theodore R. Marmor (New York: Aldine De Gruyter, 1994), 170.

6   Statistics Canada, "Socioeconomic Disparities in Birth Outcomes," November 15, 2017. Accessed at http://www.statcan.gc.ca/daily-quotidien /171115/dq171115b-eng.htm on November 15, 2017.

7   Richard S. Liu et al., "Socioeconomic Position Is Associated with Carotid Intima-Media Thickness in Mid-Childhood: The Longitudinal Study of Australian Children," *JAHA*, 2017 doi:10.1161/JAHA.117.005925

8   American Heart Association, "Disadvantaged Kids May Be at Higher Risk for Heart Disease Later in Life," *Science Daily*. Accessed at www. sciencedaily.com/releases/2017/08/170809161743.htm on August 18, 2017.

9   Centers for Disease Control and Prevention, "About the CDC-Kaiser ACE Study." Accessed at https://www.cdc.gov/violenceprevention/acestudy/ about.html on September 3, 2017.

10 Statistics Canada, *Parent-Child Associations for Physical Activity and Weight and Projected Body Mass Index*, June 21, 2017. Accessed at http:// www.statcan.gc.ca/daily-quotidien/170621/dq170621a-eng.htm on June 21, 2017.

11 Statistics Canada, *Health Reports: "Physical Activity and Sedentary Behaviour of Canadian Children Aged Three to Five,"* September 21, 2016.

12 Dave McGinn, "Canadian Children Finish 19th in 'Beep' Test," *The Globe and Mail*, September 23, 2016, L5.

13 Canadian Institute for Health Information, *Children Vulnerable in Areas of Early Development: A Determinant of Child Health*, October 2014. Accessed at https://secure.cihi.ca/free_products/Children_Vulnerable _in_Areas_of_Early_Development_EN.pdf on August 15, 2017.

14 Sharon Kirkey, "One in Four Toddlers Too Fat," *National Post*, September 29, 2016, A1.

15 R. Santos et al., *The Early Development Instrument (EDI) in Manitoba: Linking Socioeconomic Adversity and Biological Vulnerability at Birth to*

Children's Outcomes at Age 5 (Winnipeg, MB: Manitoba Centre for Health Policy, May 2012).

16   James J. Heckman, "Lead Essay: Promoting Social Mobility," *Boston Review*, September/October 2012. Accessed at http://bostonreview.net /archives/BR37.5/ndf_james_heckman_social_mobility.php on August 25, 2017.

17   Representative for Children and Youth, *Broken Promises: Alex's Story*, February 2017.

18   Marvin Shaffer, Lynell Anderson and Allison Nelson, *Opportunities in Transition: An Economic Analysis of Investing in Youth Aging out of Foster Care*, Simon Fraser University School of Public Policy. Accessed at http://www.fosteringchange.ca/opportunities_in_transition_out_now on October 18, 2016.

19   Canadian Press, "Foster Children Counted in Canadian Census for 1st Time." Accessed at http://www.cbc.ca/news/canada/foster-children -counted-in-canadian-census-for-1st-time-1.1137081 on September 24, 2017.

20   Bengt Petersson, Rodrigo Mariscal and Kotaro Ishi, *Women Are Key for Future Growth: Evidence from Canada* (International Monetary Fund, 2017).

21   BC Poverty Reduction Coalition, "Renowned Children's Advocate in Vancouver to Highlight Children's Inequality in Canada and British Columbia." Received January 16, 2017, by email. Also available at: http://bcpovertyreduction.ca/2017/01/renowned-childrens-advocate -in-vancouver-to-highlight-childrens-inequality-in-canada-and-british -columbia/

22   Lori Culbert, "Child Poverty 'a Shock' Here, UNICEF Chief Says," *Vancouver Sun*, January 17, 2017, A4.

23   First Call: BC Child and Youth Advocacy Coalition, *2016 BC Child Poverty Report Card*, November 2016.

24   Kerris Cooper and Kitty Stewart, *Does Money Affect Children's Outcomes? An Update*. Accessed at http://sticerd.lse.ac.uk/case/_new/ research/money_matters/report.asp on August 1, 2017.

25   M. Cancian, Y. Mi-Youn and K. Shook Slack, "The Effect of Additional Child Support Income on the Risk of Child Maltreatment," *Social Service Review*, 2013, 87(3): 417–437.

26 Kerris Cooper and Kitty Stewart, "Does Money Affect Children's Outcomes? An Update."

27 Kevin Milligan and Mark Stabile, "Do Child Tax Benefits Affect the Well-Being of Children? Evidence from Canadian Child Benefit Expansions," *American Economic Journal*: Economic Policy, 2011, 3: 175–205.

28 James J. Heckman, "Lead Essay: Promoting Social Mobility."

29 Mike Rose, "Response: Education and Money," *Boston Review*, September/October 2012. Accessed at http://bostonreview.net/archives/BR37.5/ndf_mike_rose_social_mobility.php on September 24, 2017.

30 Angus Reid Institute, "Kids in Canada: falling behind? Study indicates concern youth aren't getting the support they need," November 16, 2016. Accessed at www.angusreid.org/children on July 20, 2017.

CHAPTER 10

1 Martin, *Better Now*, 189.

2 Evelyn Forget, "Reconsidering a Guaranteed Annual Income: Lessons from MINCOME," *Public Sector Digest: Economics and Finance*, October 2015. Accessed at www.publicsectordigest.com/articles/view/1506 on July 19, 2017.

3 Accessed at http://brookfieldinstitute.ca/research-analysis/automation/ on August 28, 2017.

4 Accessed at https://uwaterloo.ca/canadian-index-wellbeing/reports/2016-canadian-index-wellbeing-national-report/executive-summary on September 2, 2017.

5 Statistics Canada, *Household Income in Canada: Key Results from the 2016 Census*, September 13, 2017. Accessed at http://www.statcan.gc.ca/daily-quotidien/170913/dq170913a-eng.htm on September 24, 2017.

6 Statistics Canada, *Consumer Price Index, Historical Summary (1997 to 2016)*. Accessed at http://www.statcan.gc.ca/tables-tableaux/sum-som/l01/cst01/econ46a-eng.htm on September 24, 2017.

7 Erika Dyck, "Fight Poverty to Improve Mental-Health Care," *The Globe and Mail*, May 8, 2017, A11.

8 Peter Hicks, *Toward a New Balance in Social Policy: The Future Role of Guaranteed Annual Income within the Safety Net* (C.D. Howe Institute,

January 2017). Accessed at https://www.cdhowe.org/sites/default/files/attachments/research_papers/mixed/Commentary_465_0.pdf on August 10, 2017.

9 Peter Hicks, "We're Beyond 'Basic Income' Now," *National Post*, February 8, 2017, FP9.

10 British Columbia Ministry of Finance, *Budget 2017 Update 2017/18-2019/20*, September 11, 2017, 109.

11 Accessed at https://uwaterloo.ca/canadian-index-wellbeing/reports /2016-canadian-index-wellbeing-national-report/executive-summary on September 2, 2016.

12 Canadian Institute for Health Information, *Trends in Income-Related Health Inequalities in Canada: Summary Report*, November 2015. Accessed at https://www.cihi.ca/en/summary_report_inequalities _2015_en.pdf

13 Stephen Dale, "Addressing the Social Causes of Illness," International Development Research Centre. Accessed at https://www.idrc.ca/en/ article/addressing-social-causes-illness on July 24, 2017.

14 Ben Barr, James Higgerson and Margaret Whitehead, "Investigating the Impact of the English Health Inequalities," *British Medical Journal*, 2017, 358:j3310.

15 Crawford Kilian, "'Why Austerity Kills': New Book Reveals the Human Cost of Budget Cuts," *The Tyee*, July 2, 2013. Accessed at https://thetyee. ca/Books/2013/07/02/Austerity-Kills/ on August 23, 2017.

16 Mikkonen and Raphael, *Social Determinants of Health*.

CHAPTER 11

1 Jane Philpott, "CMA Speech."

2 "Health Equity and the Social Determinants of Health," Canadian Medical Association. Accessed at https://www.cma.ca/En/Pages/health -equity.aspx on August 29, 2017.

3 Canadian Medical Association, *Health Care in Canada: What Makes Us Sick?* July 2013. Accessed at https://www.cma.ca/Assets/assets -library/document/fr/advocacy/What-makes-us-sick_en.pdf on August 25, 2017.

4   Dennis Raphael, "Addressing the Social Determinants of Health in Canada: Bridging the Gap Between Research Findings and Public Policy," *Policy Options*, March 2003, 35–40.

5   Dennis Raphael and Ambreen Sayani, "Assuming Policy Responsibility for Health Equity: Local Public Health Action in Ontario, Canada," *Health Promotion International*, (not yet published, received from author by email).

6   Linden Farrer et al., "Advocacy for Health Equity: A Synthesis Review," *The Milbank Quarterly*, 93.2 (2015): 392–437, PMC. Web. 24 September 2017.

7   Jonathan Lomas and André-Pierre Contandriopoulos, "Regulating Limits to Medicine: Towards Harmony in Public- and Self-Regulation," *Why are Some People Healthy and Others Not? The Determinants of Health of Populations*, eds. Robert G. Evans, Morris L. Barer and Theodore R. Marmor (New York: Aldine De Gruyter, 1994).

8   Accessed at https://pm.gc.ca/eng/minister-crown-indigenous-relations -and-northern-affairs-mandate-letter on August 23, 2017.

9   Accessed at http://pm.gc.ca/eng/minister-families-children-and-social -development-mandate-letter on August 23, 2017.

10   Accessed at http://pm.gc.ca/eng/minister-infrastructure-and -communities-mandate-letter on August 23, 2017.

11   *2017 Confidence and Supply Agreement between the BC Green Caucus and the BC New Democrat Caucus* (Victoria, BC: June, 2017).

12   Accessed at https://www.leg.bc.ca/documents-data/debate-transcripts /41st-parliament/2nd-session/20171017pm-CommitteeA-Blues on October 18, 2017.

13   Trevor Hancock, "Public Health and the New B.C. Government," *Times Colonist*, August 2, 2017, A8.

14   Kevin Page and Tina Yuan, "How Budget 2018 Can Reduce Poverty and Homelessness," *The Globe and Mail*, August 28, 2017, B4.

CHAPTER 12

1   Statistics Canada, "Mortality: Overview, 2012 and 2013," July 12, 2017. Accessed at http://www.statcan.gc.ca/daily-quotidien/170712/dq170712b -eng.htm on July 12, 2017.

2   Clyde Hertzman, John Frank and Robert Evans, "Heterogeneities in Health Status and the Determinants of Population Health," *Why Are Some People Healthy and Others Not? The Determinants of Health of Populations*, eds. Robert G. Evans, Morris L. Barer and Theodore R. Marmor (New York: Aldine De Gruyter, 1994).

3   Statistics Canada, *Mortality: Overview, 2012 and 2013*.

4   Vasilis Kontis et al., "Future Life Expectancy in 35 Industrialised Countries: Projections with a Bayesian Model Ensemble," *The Lancet*, February 21, 2017. Accessed at http://www.thelancet.com/journals/lancet/article/PIIS0140-6736(16)32381-9/abstract on August 25, 2017.

5   Maria Cheng, "In Wealthier Countries, Life Expectancy to Keep Rising," *Times Colonist*, February 23, 2017, D4.

6   Ryan Meili, *A Healthy Society*.

7   Canadian Public Health Association, *Public Health: A Conceptual Framework*, 2nd edition, March 2017. Accessed at https://www.cpha.ca/sites/default/files/uploads/policy/ph-framework/phcf_e.pdf on August 31, 2017.

8   Accessed at http://www.who.int/about/mission/en/ on June 15, 2017.

9   United Nations, *Universal Declaration of Human Rights*, 2015. Accessed at http://www.un.org/en/udhrbook/pdf/udhr_booklet_en_web.pdf on September 4, 2017.

10   Canadian Public Health Association, *Early Childhood Education and Care*, June 2016. Accessed at https://www.cpha.ca/sites/default/files/assets/policy/ecec_e.pdf on September 2, 2017.

11   Paul Farmer, *Pathologies of Power*, 7.

12   Wei-Ching Chang and Joy H. Fraser, "Cooperate! A Paradigm Shift for Health Equity," *International Journal for Equity in Health*, 2017. 16:12 doi:10.1186/s12939-016-0508-4. Accessed at https://equityhealthj.biomedcentral.com/articles/10.1186/s12939-016-0508-4 on July 21, 2017.

13   Ryan Meili, "Gabor Maté."

Acknowledgments

Having spent a significant amount of time thinking about what it is that gives people the best chances of being healthy, I first have to thank my parents for the good start they gave me in life. Any hope of mine as an adult to string words and thoughts together into a coherent whole has something to do with your providing a nurturing environment, reading to me and keeping the adverse experiences to a minimum. Thanks as well for the encouragement and discussion of this project, and to my dad in particular for the box of reports and other research material.

Thank you to Douglas & McIntyre for saying "yes" while this idea was still thin, to editor Pam Robertson for guiding me in focusing and improving the manuscript, and to Anna Comfort O'Keeffe, Peter Robson, Nicola Goshulak, Shed Simas, Patricia Wolfe, Setareh Ashrafologhalai and the rest of the team for seeing it through to completion. Any errors or omissions that remain are of course mine and mine alone.

The adjudicators and funder of the 2016 George Ryga Award for Social Awareness in Literature gave me encouragement at a key time. The British Columbia Arts Council provided some financial support; there's something wonderful, and not often enough acknowledged, about living in a society where you can not only say what you want to in print, including constructively criticizing the government, but that the government will help fund you to do it. That's not to be taken for granted.

Thank you to editors Robyn Smith, Barry Link and Paul Willcocks and the rest of the gang at *The Tyee*, where some of the ideas and material that appear in this book got started.

I'm blessed with many friends who took an interest in this project and encouraged me along the way. They include Robbie Newton, Foster Griezic, Bill Eisenhauer, Stephen Winn and numerous neighbourhood dog walkers. Alan Cassels asked some key questions that helped shape the direction of the project and was a supportive force throughout. Bill Warburton pointed me in some interesting directions and challenged me in ways that made the book more pragmatic than it might otherwise have been. Sharon Keen provided a steady stream of clippings and suggestions. Many sources and contacts were also generous with their time and material.

Finally, as always, a huge thank you and unbounded love to my wife, Suzanne, who listened and gave needed feedback throughout my time working on this project, and who was the first to read the manuscript and suggest improvements. As well, thanks to our daughters, Eliza and Annie, for keeping life at home calm, restorative and fun.

Select Bibliography

The following list includes works that are quoted from or referred to in the chapters of this book. It is by no means a full list of all the reference material consulted.

Anielski, Mark. *The Economics of Happiness: Building Genuine Wealth.* Gabriola Island, BC: New Society Publishers, 2007.

Ball, David. "Scared and Spied On Under Harper, Why Child Advocate Didn't Give Up." *The Tyee,* January 29, 2016.

Barr, Ben, James Higgerson, and Margaret Whitehead. "Investigating the Impact of the English Health Inequalities." *British Medical Journal,* 2017, 358:j3310.

Bell, Warren, and Amy Lubik. "Opinion: B.C.'s Climate Plan Is a Public Health Failure." *Vancouver Sun,* September 5, 2016.

Berwick, Donald, and Andrew Hackbarth. "Eliminating Waste in US Health Care." *Journal of the American Medical Association,* 2012, 307(14):1513–1516. doi:10.1001/jama.2012.362.

Blackstock, Cindy, and Sébastien Grammond. "Reforming Child Welfare First Step toward Reconciliation: Opinion." *Toronto Star,* August 1, 2017.

Blackwell, Tom. "'This Is A Lesson': One Paragraph May Have Triggered Opioid Crisis." *National Post,* June 1, 2017, A1.

Blackwell, Tom, and Monika Warzecha. "A Country Divided." *Vancouver Sun,* May 8, 2017, N2.

Boisvert, Nick. "Overdose Calls Jump 28% but Toronto Police Still Aren't Carrying Naloxone Kits." *CBC News.* November 16, 2017.

Campbell, David J.T., Kathryn King-Shier, Brenda R. Hemmelgarn, Claudia Sanmartin, Paul E. Ronksley, Robert G. Weaver, Marcello Tonelli, Deidre Hennessy, and Braden J. Manns. "*Self-Reported Financial Barriers to*

Care Among Patients with Cardiovascular-Related Chronic Conditions."
Statistics Canada, May 2014.

Canadian Institute for Health Information. *Trends in Income-Related Health Inequalities in Canada: Summary Report.* November 2015.

Canadian Press. "Air Pollution Results in 7,700 Premature Deaths in Canada Each Year, Report Says." *CBC News*, June 1, 2017.

Cancian, M., Y. Mi-Youn, and K. Shook Slack. "The Effect of Additional Child Support Income on the Risk of Child Maltreatment." *Social Service Review* 87(3) (2013): 417–437.

Carson, George, and Wendy Levinson. "Too Many Medical Procedures on Women Aren't Necessary." *Toronto Star*, June 25, 2017.

Cassels, Alan. *Seeking Sickness: Medical Screening and the Misguided Hunt for Disease.* Vancouver, BC: Greystone Books, 2012.

Caulfield, Timothy. *The Cure for Everything.* Toronto: Penguin, 2012.

Chang, Wei-Ching, and Joy H. Fraser. "Cooperate! A Paradigm Shift for Health Equity." *International Journal for Equity in Health*, 2017. 16:12 doi:10.1186/s12939-016-0508-4.

Chapin, Dwight. "How to Treat Chronic Pain without Turning to Opioids." *The Globe and Mail*, July 6, 2017, L1.

Chartier, M., M. Brownell, L. MacWilliam, J. Valdivia, Y. Nie, O. Ekuma, C. Burchill, M. Hu, L. Rajotte, and C. Kulbaba. *The Mental Health of Manitoba's Children.* Winnipeg, MB: Manitoba Centre for Health Policy, Fall 2016.

Cheng, Maria. "In Wealthier Countries, Life Expectancy to Keep Rising." *Times Colonist*, February 23, 2017, D4.

Cohen, Ronnie. "Richest Americans Live Seven to 10 Years Longer than Poorest." *Reuters Health*, December 5, 2016.

Cooper, Kerris, and Kitty Stewart. *Does Money Affect Children's Outcomes? An Update.* http://sticerd.lse.ac.uk/case/_new/research/money_matters/report.asp (accessed August 1, 2017).

Culbert, Lori. "Child Poverty 'a Shock' Here, UNICEF Chief Says." *Vancouver Sun*, January 17, 2017, A4.

Dale, Stephen. "Addressing the Social Causes of Illness." International Development Research Centre. https://www.idrc.ca/en/article/addressing-social-causes-illness (accessed July 24, 2017).

David Suzuki Foundation and Council of Canadians. *Glass Half Empty? Year*

1 *Progress Toward Resolving Drinking Water Advisories in Nine First Nations in Ontario.* February 2017.

Davis, Devra. *The Secret History of the War on Cancer.* New York: Basic Books, 2007.

Den Boef, Anthonie. "Addicts Should Get One Chance." *Vancouver Sun,* January 4, 2017, A9.

DeRosa, Katie. "$250,000-a-Year Drug Focus of Insurance Fight." *Times Colonist,* September 22, 2017, A3.

Devlin, Hannah. "Living Near Heavy Traffic Increases Risk of Dementia, Say Scientists." *The Guardian,* January 5, 2017.

Duffy, Robert, Gaetan Royer, and Charley Beresford. *Who's Picking Up the Tab? Federal and Provincial Downloading Onto Local Governments.* Vancouver: Columbia Institute Centre for Civic Governance, September 2014.

Dyck, Erika. "Fight Poverty to Improve Mental-Health Care." *The Globe and Mail,* May 8, 2017, A11.

Eagland, Nick. "First Nations People Three Times More Likely to Die from Overdose, Stats Show." *Vancouver Sun,* August 4, 2017, A8.

Egen, Olivia, et al. "Health and Social Conditions of the Poorest Versus Wealthiest Counties in the United States." *American Journal of Public Health,* December 7, 2016.

Epp, J. *Achieving Health for All: A Framework for Health Promotion.* Ottawa: Health and Welfare Canada, 1986.

Evans, Robert G., Morris L. Barer and Theodore R. Marmor, eds. *Why Are Some People Healthy and Others Not? The Determinants of Health of Populations.* New York, NY: Aldine De Gruyter, 1994.

Farmer, Paul. *Pathologies of Power: Health, Human Rights, and the New War on the Poor.* Berkeley, CA: University of California Press, 2003.

Farrer, Linden, et al. "Advocacy for Health Equity: A Synthesis Review." *The Milbank Quarterly,* 93.2 (2015): 392–437. PMC. Web. September 24, 2017.

Fayerman, Pamela. "Judy Darcy: 'I Will Pour My Heart and Soul' into Mental Health/Addictions File." *Vancouver Sun,* July 27, 2017.

Forget, Evelyn. "Reconsidering a Guaranteed Annual Income: Lessons from MINCOME." *Public Sector Digest: Economics and Finance.* October 2015.

Galea, Sandro. *Health in New York and Chicago by Subway and L-Stops: A Pictorial Essay.* Boston University School of Public Health, May 17, 2015.

Galloway, Gloria. "NDP Vows to Make Health Top Priority." *The Globe and*

Mail, September 8, 2016.

——. "Ottawa Still Failing to Provide Health Care on Reserves: Report." *The Globe and Mail*, January 25, 2017, A5.

Garfield, Leanna. "Food Prices Are Insanely High in Rural Canada, where Ketchup Costs $14 and Sunny D Costs $29." *Business Insider*, September 21, 2017.

Gawande, Atul. "Tell Me Where It Hurts." *New Yorker*, January 23, 2017, 36–45.

Gee, Alastair, Liz Barney, and Julia O'Malley. "How America Counts Its Homeless—and Why So Many Are Overlooked." *The Guardian*, February 16, 2017.

Goering, Paula, Scott Veldhuizen, Aimee Watson, Carol Adair, Brianna Kopp, Eric Latimer, Geoff Nelson, Eric MacNaughton, David Streiner, and Tim Aubry. *National At Home/Chez Soi Final Report*. Calgary, AB: Mental Health Commission of Canada, 2014.

Graham, Jennifer. "Chief Perry Bellegarde Opens AFN Meeting with Plea to End Racism, Violence." *The Canadian Press*, July 25, 2017.

Grant, Kelly. "Opioid Prescriptions Increasing in Ontario, Despite Crisis." *The Globe and Mail*, May 17, 2017, A3.

——. "Study Highlights Unneeded Medical Care." *The Globe and Mail*, April 7, 2017, A10.

Hager, Mike. "Ottawa Rejects Expert Calls to Decriminalize Illegal Opioids." *The Globe and Mail*, August 28, 2017, S1.

Hancock, Trevor. "Beyond Health Care: From Public Health Policy to Healthy Public Policy." *Canadian Journal of Public Health*. May/June 1985, 9–11.

——. "Public Health and the New B.C. Government." *Times Colonist*, August 2, 2017, A8.

——. "The Secret of Medicine is Masterly Inactivity." *Times Colonist*, November 16, 2016, A8.

——. "Why Did Mary Die? Dig Deep to Find Causes." *Times Colonist*, September 6, 2017, A8.

Healthy People 2000: National Health Promotion and Disease Prevention Objectives. Boston: Jones and Bartlett Publishers, 1992.

Heckman, James J. "Lead Essay: Promoting Social Mobility." *Boston Review*, September/October 2012.

Heft, David. "Mental Health-Care Services Quietly Eroding." *Times Colonist*, February 7, 2017, A11.

Herper, Matthew. "The World's Most Expensive Drugs." *Forbes*, February
22, 2010.

Hicks, Peter. *Toward a New Balance in Social Policy: The Future Role of
Guaranteed Annual Income within the Safety Net.* C.D. Howe Institute,
January 2017.

———. "We're Beyond 'Basic Income' Now" *National Post*, February 8,
2017, FP9.

Hyslop, Katie. "First Nations Still Vastly Overrepresented in BC Overdose
Deaths." *The Tyee*, August 3, 2017.

Irwin, Lori G., Arjumand Siddiqi, and Clyde Hertzman. "Early Child
Development: A Powerful Equalizer." World Health Organization's
Commission on the Social Determinants of Health, 2007.

Ivanova, Iglika. "The Cost of Poverty in BC." Canadian Centre for Policy
Alternatives, BC Office, July 2011.

Jackson, Andrew. "Beware the Canadian Austerity Model." Canadian Centre
for Policy Alternatives, June 1, 2010.

Katz, Alan, Jennifer Enns, and Kathi Avery Kinew. "Canada Needs a Holistic
First Nations Health Strategy." *Canadian Medical Association Journal*,
August 8, 2017.

Kelland, Kate. "Sperm Count Falling Sharply in Developed World,
Researchers Say." *Reuters*, July 25, 2017.

Kelly, Doug. "The Hidden Complexities in Substance Addiction." *The Globe
and Mail*, August 25, 2017, S2.

Khullar, Dhruv. "Social Isolation Is a Growing Epidemic, One That's
Increasingly Recognized as Having Dire Physical, Mental and Emotional
Consequences." *New York Times*, December 22, 2016.

Kilian, Crawford. "'Why Austerity Kills': New Book Reveals the Human Cost
of Budget Cuts." *The Tyee*, July 2, 2013.

Kirkey, Sharon. "One in Four Toddlers Too Fat." *National Post*, September 29,
2016, A1.

Kirkup, Kristy. "B.C. Officials Eye Portugal's Drug Policy." *The Globe and Mail*,
August 10, 2017, S2.

Kluge, Eike-Henner. "Health Ministry Has to Make Hard Choices." *Times
Colonist*, October 1, 2017, A11.

Knapton, Sarah. "Car Engine Particles Linked to Alzheimer's." *National Post*,
September 6, 2016, A2.

Kontis, Vasilis, et al. "Future Life Expectancy in 35 Industrialised Countries: Projections with a Bayesian Model Ensemble." *The Lancet*, February 21, 2017.

Lalonde, Marc. *A New Perspective on the Health of Canadians: A Working Document*. Ottawa: April 1974.

Lambert, Bev. "In Resolving Addiction, Address the Root Causes." *Times Colonist*, August 4, 2017, A13.

Lamontagne, Manon. *Violence Against Aboriginal Women: Scan and Report*. Canadian Women's Foundation. October 31, 2011.

Levi, Gloria, and Laura Kadawaki. *Our Future: Seniors, Socialization, and Health*. Vancouver, BC: Columbia Institute, April 2016.

Levinson, Wendy. "Over One Million Canadians Get Unneeded Tests." *The Province*, April 30, 2017, A26.

Li, Na, Naomi Dachner and Valerie Tarasuk. "The Impact of Changes in Social Policies on Household Food Insecurity in British Columbia, 2005–2012." *Preventive Medicine* 93 (2016): 151–158.

Li, Wanyee. "Mental Health and Drug Addiction included in Vancouver Police's Top Priorities." *Metro News*. metronews.ca (accessed January 24, 2017).

Liu, Richard S., Fiona K. Mensah, John Carlin, Ben Edwards, Sarath Ranganathan, Michael Cheung, Terence Dwyer, Richard Saffery, Costan G. Magnussen, Markus Juonala, Melissa Wake, and David P. Burgner. "Socioeconomic Position Is Associated With Carotid Intima-Media Thickness in Mid-Childhood: The Longitudinal Study of Australian Children." *Journal of the American Heart Association*, 2017, doi:10.1161/JAHA.117.005925.

Lovgreen, Tina. "Fears of Accidental Exposure to Fentanyl Hamper Efforts of Conservation Groups." *CBC News*, June 13, 2017.

Lupick, Travis. "B.C. Manifesto for Better Mental Health Calls for Province to Prioritize Prevention and Support in the Community." *Georgia Straight*, October 11, 2016.

———. "Vancouver Prescription Heroin Users Wage Court Battle with the Feds." *Georgia Straight*, March 19, 2014.

Martin, Danielle. *Better Now: Six Big Ideas to Improve Health Care for All Canadians*. Canada: Allen Lane, 2017.

McBain, Leslie. "My Son's Death Offers Lessons for Ending the Opioid Epidemic." *The Globe and Mail*, September 1, 2017, S1.

McElroy, Justin. "Kamloops Experiencing Worst Air Quality in Its Recorded History." *CBC News*, August 3, 2017.

McFarlane, Lawrie. "'Deaths from Despair' Demand Answers." *Times Colonist*, March 31, 2017, A11.

McGinn, Dave. "Canadian Children Finish 19th in 'Beep' Test." *The Globe and Mail*, September 23, 2016, L5.

McIntosh, Diane. "Fentanyl Scourge Tied to Mental Health Crisis." *The Province*, July 2, 2017, A21.

McQuigge, Michelle. "Many Tests on Patients a Waste of Time: Study." *Times Colonist*, April 7, 2017, C1.

Meili, Ryan. *A Healthy Society: How a Focus on Health Can Revive Canadian Democracy*. Saskatoon, SK: Purich Publishing Ltd., 2012.

———. "Gabor Maté: On Storytelling, Health, and the Ruling Class." *Briarpatch*, November 18, 2014.

Mikkonen, Juha, and Dennis Raphael. *Social Determinants of Health: The Canadian Facts*. Toronto: York University School of Health Policy and Management, 2010.

Milligan, Kevin, and Mark Stabile. "Do Child Tax Benefits Affect the Well-Being of Children? Evidence from Canadian Child Benefit Expansions." *American Economic Journal: Economic Policy* 3 (2011): 175–205.

Minsky, Amy. "First Nations 'Living in Third World Conditions' as Communities Endure Water Advisories." *Global News*, February 9, 2017.

Mittelstaedt, Martin. "Pollution Debate Born of Chemical Valley's Girl-Baby Boom." *The Globe and Mail*, November 15, 2005.

Mora, Camilo, et al. "Global Risk of Deadly Heat." *Nature Climate Change*, June 19, 2017, 7, 501–506.

Mosby, Ian, and Tracey Galloway. "'Hunger Was Never Absent': How Residential School Diets Shaped Current Patterns of Diabetes among Indigenous Peoples in Canada." *Canadian Medical Association Journal*, August 14, 2017.

O'Neil, Peter. "Mayors Link Drug Crisis, Housing Need." *Vancouver Sun*, January 21, 2017, A4.

Orwell, George. *The Road to Wigan Pier*. Harmondsworth, England: Penguin Books, 1975. (Copyright 1937.)

Page, Kevin, and Tina Yuan. "How Budget 2018 Can Reduce Poverty and Homelessness." *The Globe and Mail*, August 28, 2017, B4.

Peters, Diane. "Charismatic Guru Popularized Ancient Ideas." *The Globe and Mail*, July 29, 2017, S16.

Petersson, Bengt, Rodrigo Mariscal, and Kotaro Ishi. *Women Are Key for Future Growth: Evidence from Canada*. International Monetary Fund, 2017.

Petrescu, Sarah. "B.C. Spent $3 Million on Tent City, Papers Show." *Times Colonist*, Thursday, August 3, 2017, A1.

Philpott, Jane. "CMA Speech." Health Canada, August 21, 2017.

———. "Getting to the Root of Canada's Opioid Crisis." *The Globe and Mail*, January 16, 2017, S2.

———. "30 things I've learned in 30 years as a doctor." Dr. Jane Philpott blog, August 24, 2014.

Picard, André. *Matters of Life and Death*. Madeira Park, BC: Douglas & McIntyre, 2017.

Piver, Andre C. "Mental-Health Workers Must Be Allowed to Care, Provide Hope." *Vancouver Sun*, March 25, 2017, B4.

Potkins, Meghan. "Alberta Opioid Crisis 'Completely Out of Hand.'" *National Post*, September 5, 2017, A3.

Provincial Health Services Authority. *Priority Health Equity Indicators for British Columbia: Selected Indicators Report*. Vancouver, BC: Provincial Health Services Authority, Population and Public Health Program, 2016.

Public Health Agency of Canada. *The Direct Economic Burden of Socio-Economic Health Inequalities in Canada*. Ottawa, 2016.

Raphael, Dennis. "Addressing the Social Determinants of Health in Canada: Bridging the Gap Between Research Findings and Public Policy." *Policy Options* (March 2003): 35–40.

Raphael, Dennis, and Ambreen Sayani. "Assuming Policy Responsibility for Health Equity: Local Public Health Action in Ontario, Canada." *Health Promotion International* (not yet published, received from author by email).

Raphael, Dennis, and Toba Bryant. "Income Inequality Is Killing Thousands of Canadians Every Year." *Toronto Star*, November 23, 2014.

Representative for Children and Youth. *Too Many Victims: Sexualized Violence in the Lives of Children and Youth in Care*. Victoria, BC: October 2016.

Rose, Mike. "Response: Education and Money." *Boston Review*, September/October 2012.

Santos, R., M. Brownell, O. Ekuma, T. Mayer, and R. Soodeen. *The Early Development Instrument (EDI) in Manitoba: Linking Socioeconomic Adversity and Biological Vulnerability at Birth to Children's Outcomes at Age 5*. Winnipeg, MB: Manitoba Centre for Health Policy, May 2012.

Schneider, Eric C., Dana O. Sarnak, David Squires, Arnav Shah, and Michelle M. Doty. *Mirror, Mirror 2017: International Comparison Reflects Flaws and Opportunities for Better U.S. Health Care*. The Commonwealth Fund, July 2017.

Semeniuk, Ivan. "Scientists Calculate Rising Risk of Lethal Heat Waves." *The Globe and Mail*, June 20, 2017, A4.

Shaffer, Marvin, Lynell Anderson, and Allison Nelson. *Opportunities in Transition: An Economic Analysis of Investing in Youth Aging out of Foster Care*. Simon Fraser University School of Public Policy. http://www.fosteringchange.ca/opportunities_in_transition_out_now on (accessed October 18, 2016).

Sherlock, Tracy. "Cindy Blackstock Says Trudeau Government's 'Making Excuses' for Neglecting Indigenous Children." *National Observer*, July 31, 2017.

Shingler, Benjamin. "Sarnia Area First Nation Facing Health Problems from Exposure to Pollutants." *Toronto Star* (The Canadian Press), November 24, 2013.

Shore, Randy. "Cost a Factor in Filling Drug Prescriptions." *Vancouver Sun*, February 2, 2017, A7.

Simpson, Jeffrey. *Chronic Condition: Why Canada's Health-Care System Needs to Be Dragged into the 21st Century*. Toronto: Allen Lane, 2012.

Slaughter, Graham. "Canadian Doctor Shows Off Her Health Card at Bernie Sanders' Medicare Bill Launch." *CTV News*, September 13, 2017.

Smolina, Kate, and Kim Rutherford. "Alternatives to Opioids Needed for Chronic Pain Relief." *The Province*, January 30, 2017, A15.

So, Linda. "Ohio County Claims Top Spot in America's Opioid Death Spiral." *Reuters*, June 21, 2017.

Springmann, Marco, et al. "Global and Regional Health Effects of Future Food Production under Climate Change: A Modelling Study." *The Lancet*, volume 387, issue 10031, 1937–1946.

Stanbrook, Matthew. "Why the Federal Government Must Lead in Health Care." *Canadian Medical Association Journal*, August 17, 2015.

St. Denis, Jen. "Overdose Crisis Affecting Vancouver's Indigenous at Stunningly High Rate: Chief Medical Officer." *Metro News*. metronews.ca (accessed July 26, 2017).

Sterritt, Angela. "Indigenous Kids Largely Apprehended because of Poverty, Says Former Child Protection Worker." *CBC News*, November 21, 2017.

Temple, Norman J. and Andrew Thompson. *Exce$$ive Medical $pending: Facing the Challenge*. Oxford: Radcliffe Publishing, 2007.

Theman, Trevor. "How Doctors Can Stop Making Opioid Addicts." *The Globe and Mail*, April 8, 2017, S3.

Tieleman, Bill. "Drug Overdoses Kill Four a Day in BC, and Inaction and Apathy Are to Blame." *The Tyee*, July 11, 2017.

Tjepkema, Michael, Russell Wilkins, and Andrea Long. *Cause-Specific Mortality by Income Adequacy in Canada: A 16-Year Follow-Up Study*. Statistics Canada. http://www.statcan.gc.ca/pub/82-003-x/2013007/article/11852-eng.htm (accessed August 14, 2017).

Todd, Douglas. "Fentanyl: A Men's Health Crisis." *Vancouver Sun*, March 20, 2017.

Tupper, Kenneth. "How to Stem Overdose Cases." *Vancouver Sun*, August 12, 2017, B2.

Verbrugge, Isolde. "Consumption Sites Not About Wellness." *Times Colonist*, August 20, 2017, A11.

Wakefield, Jonny. "'What's in That Fish?' Scientists Set to Launch Major Study of Mercury in Williston Lake." *Dawson Creek Mirror*, May 27, 2016.

Wilkinson, Richard, and Kate Pickett. *The Spirit Level: Why Equality is Better for Everyone*. London: Penguin Books, 2009.

Wong, Jackie. "An Urgent Call on Overdose Crisis: Prescribe Drugs, End Prohibition." *The Tyee*, January 26, 2017.

———. "In Throes of Overdose Crisis, a Community Unites to Fight Back." *The Tyee*, January 1, 2017.

———. "The Overdose Crisis: We Know How to Save Lives, Doctors Say." *The Tyee*, January 27, 2017.

Woo, Andrea. "Overdose Rate Higher among First Nations." *The Globe and Mail*, Friday, August 4, 2017, A4.

Wood, Evan. "Opioid Crisis Calls for Smarter Prescribing." *The Globe and Mail*, July 27, 2017, S2.

Index

Page numbers in **bold** refer to figures.

Aboriginal Head Start on Reserve program, 124

Aboriginal health. *See* Indigenous health in Canada

Aboriginal Homelessness Steering Committee, 115

Adams, Evan, 129, 130

addiction, 86–88, 90–91, 92, 94
  as health issue, 97, 101, 145
  socioeconomic factors, 100, 105
  underlying causes, 106–7, 110, 111
  See also opioid crisis

Adverse Childhood Experiences (ACE) study, 149

air pollution, 124–25, 139

Alexander, Bruce, 110–11

American Journal of Public Health, 64

Anderson, Lynell, 157

Angl, Emily Nicholas, 36–37

Angus Reid Institute, 162

Azeez, Lina, 99

Balay-Karperien, Audrey, 56

Baranyai, Zeb, 79–80, 84

Barer, Morris, 20, 51

Barnes, Constance, 100

Barton, Curtis, 69

basic income, 164–68, 170

Basu, Niladri, 140

Basu, Sanjay, 174

Baum, Fran, 179

BC Centre for Disease Control Operations and Chronic Disease Prevention, 68, 105

BC Centre on Substance Use, 103, 104

BC Civil Liberties Association, 73

BC Housing, 92

BC Medical Association, 42

Bégin, Monique, 29, 30

Bellegarde, Perry, 113

Bellringer, Carol, 52, 53–54

Bennett, Carolyn, 185

Beresford, Charley, 88

Better Now (book), 146, 164

Bilsker, Dan, 108

Blackstock, Cindy, 121–22, 123, 157

Bloch, Gary, 71–72

Body Economic, The (book), 174

Brem, Mike, 98

Brend, Yvette, 81

British Medical Journal (BMJ), 50, 172, 173

Broken Promises (report), 156

Brooks-Lim, Elizabeth, 96–97

Bryant, Toba, 77

Building on Values (report), 178

Canada Child Tax Benefit, 158

Canada Health Act, 43

Canada Health Action (report), 23

Canadian Association of Physicians for the Environment, 140

Canadian Cancer Society, 47

Canadian Community Health Survey, 75

Canadian Doctors for Medicare, 165

Canadian Federation of Nurses Unions, 43

Canadian Health Coalition, 42, 43

Canadian Health Measures Survey, 151

Canadian Index of Wellbeing, 167, 170

Canadian Institute for Health Information (CIHI), 26–27, 28, 46, 48, 49, 50, 153, 170–71

Canadian Medical Association, 38, 41, 71, 124, 176, 177, 178

Canadian Medical Association Journal (CMAJ), 37, 41, 117, 131, 152

Canadian Mental Health Association, 80, 81, 82, 93

Canadian Population Health Initiative, 141

Canadian Public Health Association (CPHA), 143, 144, 190, 191–92

Canadian Women's Foundation, 114

cancer, 26, 47–48, 58

cardiovascular disease, 13–14, 26

Carson, George, 46

Cassels, Alan, 47

Caulfield, Timothy, 16, 72

Centers for Disease Control and Prevention, 26, 98, 103, 149

Centre for Nursing and Health Studies, 58

Chang, Wei-Ching, 192

Chapin, Dwight, 102

Charleson, April, 119, 120

Chen, Hong, 139

childbirth and maternity care, 46–47

Children First Canada, 162

children's health
  adverse experiences, 24, 145–46, **150, 151, 154, 155**
  and education, 158
  and income, 146, 148, 149, 152, 154, 159, 160–62
  and positive factors, 147, 155

Choosing Wisely Canada, 46, 48, 49

Chronic Condition (book), 60

Clark, Christy, 91

climate change and health, 135–36, 137, 143

Coleman, Rich, 91

Commission on Social
    Determinants of Health,
    29, 76
Common Drug Review, 58
Commonwealth Fund, 35, 39, 42, 71
Contandriopoulos, André-Pierre,
    183–84
Cooper, Kerris, 160, 161
Copas, Lorraine, 70
Copes, Ray, 139
Costs of Pollution in Canada
    (report), 138
Council of Canadians, 141
Cure for Everything, The (book)
    16, 72

Daly, Patricia, 112
Dartmouth Atlas of Health Care,
    49–50
David Suzuki Foundation, 141
Davies, Don, 43
Davis, Devra, 142
Day, Brian, 35
Decter, Michael, 37–38
dementia, 139, 140
Dennis, Conrad, 70
dentistry, 45
diabetes, 14, **15**, 118, **127**
Diabetes Canada, 14
diet and health, 15, 74–75
Dingwall, David, 23
Dix, Adrian, 58, 187
Dora, Carlos, 139, 143
Drasic, Lydia, 68
Drug Benefit Council, 58
drug spending, 40, 56–58

Duclos, Yves, 186
Duncan, John, 120
Dyck, Erika, 167–68

Enns, Jennifer, 131, 132
environmental causes of illness,
    134–44. *See also* air
    pollution; climate change
    and health; extreme
    weather events; forest fires
Epp, Jake, 21, 22, 23, 26
Evans, Mike, 36
Evans, Robert, 20, 51, 148, 189
Exce$$ive Medical $pending (book),
    51, 56
extreme weather events, 136–37. *See
    also* forest fires
Ezzati, Majid, 189

Fairness for Children (report), 158
Family Unification Program, 123
Farmer, Paul, 192
fentanyl, 96, 97, 98, 99, 100, 104. *See
    also* opioid crisis
First Call: BC Child and Youth
    Advocacy Coalition, 159
First Nations Child and Family
    Caring Society (FNCFCS),
    120, 121, 157
First Nations health. *See* Indigenous
    health in Canada
*First Nations Health and Well-Being
    Interim Update*, 125
First Nations Health Authority
    (FNHA), 112, 113, 116, 125,
    128, 129

First Nations Health Council, 112, 114, 145

food insecurity, 72–73, 117, 178

Food Secure Canada, 119

forest fires, 134–36

Forget, Evelyn, 165

foster care, 156–57

Flanders, Dan, 152–53

fracking, 140

Frank, Johan Peter, 190

Frank, John, 171, 189

Fraser, Joy, 58, 192

Fry, Hedy, 42

Galloway, Gloria, 124

Galloway, Tracey, 117, 118

Gauvin, Emma, 69

Gawande, Atul, 55

Gervais, Alex, 155–56, 157

government, Canadian
    health care spending, 28–29
    role in health reform, 18, 19, 37, 39, 40–41, 42, 178, 180–81

Grammond, Sébastien, 122

Grantham, Sarah, 79, 84

Hancock, Trevor, 19–20, 50, 187

Harcourt, Mike, 182, 183

Hawryluk, Ted, 73

Health Care in Canada (report), 177

health care system in Canada, 11
    challenges, 21
    health transfer payments, 41, 44, 61
    inaccessibility, 36–37, 49

international comparisons, 35–36

and national pride, 34, 40

and preventive care, 52, 53, 54, 58–59

and private care, 34, 52

spending, 19, **36**, 39, 43, 44, 51, 52, 54–55, 60–61

wasted funds, 45, 46, 49, 50, 52

See also pharmaceutical coverage in Canada

Health Promotion International, 179

Healthy People 2000 (Sullivan report), 24–26

Healthy Society, A (book), 61

Heart and Stroke Foundation of Canada, 13

heart disease, 26, 58

Heckman, James, 162

Heft, David, 81

Helps, Lisa, 89

Henry, Bonnie, 135

Hertzman, Clyde, 146, 188

Hicks, Peter, 168

Hodge, Matthew, 148

homelessness, 85–88, 90–91, 93, 110, 178

Horgan, John, 91, 92, 93, 100, 164

Hoskins, Eric, 193

housing costs, 70, 107

Hulchanski, David, 70

Human Early Learning Partnership, 146

Hungry for Justice (report), 73

Indigenous Health Alliance, 124
Indigenous health in Canada
    addiction, 110, 111, 115
    diabetes, 118, **127**
    healthcare on reserves, 124
    homelessness, 89–90, 115
    inequality and discrimination,
        38, 93, 113, 120, 121, 125,
        126–27, **128**, 129, 141, 177
    malnourishment, 118–19
    mental health and suicide,
        114, 116
    poverty, 116, 117, 120, 121, 131
    self-governance, 122, 127,
        128, 132
    trauma, 112, 113, 115, 122, 129,
        130, 131, 145, 156
    violence, 113–14, 116, 130
    See also residential schools
individualism and health, 13, 14, 21,
    23, 25, 31, 180
inequality and health, 10, 22, 27
    cost, 61, 68, 166
    by gender, 68, 108
    by income, 67, 68, **77**
    and lifestyle, 72–75
    reducing inequality, 28
    by region, 63–64, 67
    role of material hardship, 69–70
    role of social status, 74–76
Institute for Clinical Evaluative
    Sciences, 139
Institute of Population and Public
    Health, 171–72
International Development
    Research Centre, 171

International Health Policy Survey
    of Older Adults, 71
International Institute for
    Sustainable Development
    (IISD), 138
International Journal for Equity in
    Health, 192
In the Realm of Hungry Ghosts
    (book), 107
Irwin, Lori, 146
Island Health, 81
isolation and health, 82–83, 107, 111

Jackson, Andrew, 24
Jang, Kerry, 90–91
Jansen, Brandon Juhani, 106
Jewell, Nicholas, 86
Journal of the American Heart
    Association, 149
Journal of the American Medical
    Association, 49

Kadawaki, Laura, 83
Katz, Alan, 131, 132
Kelly, Doug, 112, 145
Kendall, Perry, 127–28, 163
Khullar, Dhruv, 82–83
Kilian, Crawford, 174
Kinew, Kathi Avery, 131, 132
Kluge, Eike-Henner, 58
Knott, Helen, 118–19, 130, 131

Lafontaine, Alika, 124
Lake, Terry, 101
Lalonde, Marc, 17–19

Lalonde report, 17–19, 20, 21, 23, 26, 32, 45, 194

Lambert, Bev, 114, 115

Lamontagne, Manon, 114

Lapointe, Lisa, 96, 99

Levi, Gloria, 83

Levinson, Wendy, 46, 47, 48, 49

Lexchin, Joel, 56

Liberal Party of Canada, 31, 42, 88, 179–80, 185

lifestyle and health, 14–15, 20–21, 58–59, 74–75, 165–66, 180

Liu, Richard, 149

Lomas, Jonathan, 183–84

loneliness. *See* isolation and health

MacKendrick, Andrew, 101

Maher, Barbara, 139

Manitoba Centre for Health Policy, 154

Marmor, Theodore, 20, 51

Marmot, Michael, 28, 75–76

Martin, Danielle, 34, 146, 164, 165

Maté, Gabor, 107, 193

Matters of Life and Death (book), 61, 93

May, Theresa, 173

McBain, Leslie, 100

McDonald, Shannon, 113, 116

McFarlane, Lawrie, 107–8

McIntosh, Diane, 110

medical error, 50–51

Medical Society Consortium on Climate and Health (MSCCH), 136, 137

Medicare Protection Act, 35

Meili, Ryan, 61

Mental Health Act, 94

mental illness

difficulty accessing care, 79–83, 92

as health care priority, 23, 45, 93, 107, 177

and health inequity, 66

needed reforms, 110

underlying issues, 23, 89, 91, 93, 109, 110, 136

Meredith, John, 135

Mikkonen, Juha, 28–29, 72, 174–75

Milligan, Kevin, 161–62

Mora, Camilo, 137

Morgan, Steve, 71

Morley, David, 158, 159

Morris, Jonny, 82

Mosby, Ian, 117, 118

Mustard, Fraser, 28

My Health My Community (survey), 66

National Housing Strategy, 88, 186

Natural Resources Canada, 135

Naylor, David, 39–40, 41, 44

New Deal, 174

New England Journal of Medicine, 59

New Perspective on the Health of Canadians, A (Lalonde report), 17–19, 20, 21, 23, 26, 32

Niwe, Ronin (Dave), 110

Nutrition North, 185

Nutt, Samantha, 62, 193, 194

obesity, 26, 27, 52, 150, 152

opioid crisis, 89, 98, 99

    management of, 101–2, 104, 106, 186

    overdose deaths, 95–97, 107, 177

    role of prescription opioids, 103, 104, 105, 106

    See also fentanyl

Opportunities in Transition (report), 157

Organisation for Economic Co-operation and Development (OECD), 29, 42

Overdose Prevention Society, 100

overtreatment, 46–51

Palmer, Adam, 106

Paterson, Neil, 80

Patients Canada, 36, 38

Peach, Derek, 95, 100–1

Pelerine, J. Gary, 16–17

Perry, Tom, 56–57, 182, 183

Petrovich, Curt, 81

PharmaCare, 57

pharmaceutical coverage in Canada, 37–38, 42, 43, 45, 71

Philpott, Jane, 31, 32, 101, 106, 107, 124, 125, 176–77, 178, 185

Picard, André, 61, 93

Pickett, Kate, 73–74

Pierre, Sophie, 133

Piver, Andre, 109

Pless, Barry, 148

Portman, Stephen, 86

Provincial Health Services Authority, 67–68

Public Health Agency of Canada, 61–62

Public Health Ontario, 139

racism and health, 113, 114–15. *See also* inequity and discrimination *under* Indigenous health in Canada

Rankin, Murray, 96

Raphael, Dennis, 14, 28–29, 32, 72, 77, 115, 174–75, 179–80

Read, Nicole, 87–88, 89–90

Regional Homelessness Task Force, 93

residential schools, 117, 118, 119, 121, 123, 129, 130

Richard, Bernard, 155, 156

Roadmap to Men's Health, A (report), 108

Robertson, Gregor, 107

Robert Wood Johnson Foundation, 64

Romanow, Roy, 178–79, 181

Rose, Mike, 162

Royal Commission on Aboriginal Peoples, 114

Royal Commission on the Future of Healthcare in Canada, 178

Ruble, Norm, 85–87, 92, 98

Rutherford, Kim, 105

screening, 46–49, 53, 55–56

Secret History of the War on Cancer, The (book), 142

Seeking Sickness (book), 47

Semmelweis, Ignaz, 190

Sen, Amartya, 66

Shaffer, Marvin, 157

Shand, Christianna, 80

Shay, Christopher, 69–70

Siddiqi, Arjumand, 146

Silnicki, Adrienne, 43

Simpson, Chris, 38, 39

Simpson, Jeffrey, 60

smoking, 16–17, 27, 28, 75, 143, 171

Smolina, Kate, 105

social determinants of health, 11, 16, 17, 18, 32, 60, 177

Social Determinants of Health (book), 72, 174

Social Development Canada, 168

Sohi, Amarjeet, 186

sperm count declines, 138

Spirit Level, The (book), 73

Stabile, Mark, 161–62

Stanbrook, Matthew, 37

Stewart, Kitty, 160, 161

Stone, Michael, 104

STOP HIV/AIDS (program), 69

Stuckler, David, 174

Sullivan, Louis W., 24–25

Tam, Theresa, 101

Temple, Norman, 51, 54, 55–56, 60

tent cities, 84–88, 89, 91, 94, 98, 99, 110, 115

Therapeutics Initiative, 57

Thompson, Andrew, 51, 54, 55–56

Tjepkema, Michael, 77

Together Against Poverty Society, 86

Toronto Health Profiles, 63

Transformative Change Accord: First Nations Health Plan, 125

Trends in Income-Related Health Inequalities in Canada (report), 170

Trudeau, Justin, 31, 32, 42, 43, 107, 178, 179–80, 185

Truth and Reconciliation Commission, 118, 122, 130

Tupper, Kenneth, 104

Turpel-Lafond, Mary Ellen, 157

2015 federal election, 31, 41, 43

2014 National Climate Assessment, 143

Tyers, Stacey, 69

UNICEF Canada, 158

Union of British Columbia Municipalities (UBCM), 87, 89

United Nations Convention on the Rights of the Child, 191

United Nations Declaration on the Rights of Indigenous People, 186

Universal Declaration of Human Rights, 191

US Department of Health and Human Services, 24